Top 10 Truths About Vaccinations
You Don't Know, What You Don't Know

Dr. Scott G. McLeod

Copyright © 2025 by Scott G. McLeod, D.C.

No part of this publication may be reproduced, stored in a retrieval system, or transmitted in any form or by any means—electronic, mechanical, photocopying, recording, or otherwise—without the prior written permission of the author, except in the case of brief quotations embodied in critical articles or reviews.

ISBN: 979-8-218-76909-3

Published by Open Eye Media, LLC

This book is a work of non-fiction. While every effort has been made to ensure the accuracy and reliability of the information provided, the author makes no representations or warranties with respect to the completeness or accuracy of the contents and specifically disclaims any implied warranties of fitness for a particular purpose.

This book is not intended as medical advice and should not be used as a substitute for consulting a licensed healthcare provider. The views expressed are those of the author and do not necessarily reflect those of any institution or professional body.

Printed in the United States of America
First Edition

The views in this book are rooted in the laws of nature, science, and human physiology. They reflect the perspectives of independent, unbiased doctors and scientists from around the world—voices not owned, sponsored, or silenced by industry interests.

It is not recommended that you alter your medical care without the knowledge of your healthcare advisor.

It is, however, strongly recommended that you take ownership of your health—and the health of your children—so you can make truly informed decisions for your family, and find a healthcare advisor who respects your right to think for yourself.

The views of this book may not match the views of the AMA, CDC, FDA, AAP, WHO, or Big Pharma—because I'm not on their payroll.

Dedication

To my father —
At a time when vaccinating children was considered the unquestionable norm, he had the wisdom to seek truth over tradition. While others followed blindly, he educated himself. When the world around him bowed to medical pressure, he stood firmly in his convictions. He chose a path few dared to walk — guided not by fear or conformity, but by knowledge, courage, and vision.

To my mother —
Your bravery to trust in my father's discernment was an act of quiet strength. Together, you made a choice that defied the expectations of your time — not out of rebellion, but out of love and hope for a healthier future.

Because of your sacrifices, I have the healthy unvaccinated life I live today. Because of your strength, I began the journey that led me to research, question, and uncover the deeper truths behind one of the most important issues of our time.

With deepest gratitude and love.

Table of Contents

Chapter 1: The Thinking Behind the Science   16

Chapter 2: Truth #1 - The Entire Vaccine Model Is Built on a Faulty Assumption   26

Chapter 3: Immunology 101   49

Chapter 4: Truth #2 - Vaccines Don't Build Herd Immunity—They Undermine It   82

Chapter 5: Truth #3 - Vaccines Didn't Save Us from Disease—We Were Already Winning   95

Chapter 6: Truth #4 - The "Safe and Effective" Mantra Is a Marketing Line—Not Science   128

Chapter 7: Risks vs. Benefits   225

Chapter 8: Truth #5 - Vaccines Can—and Do—Cause Serious Harm   303

Chapter 9: Truth #6 - There's Big Money Behind Every Shot   322

Chapter 10: Truth #7 - Your Doctor Is Supposed to Tell You More—They Usually Don't   344

Chapter 11: Truth #8 - Public School Does Not Require Vaccination—Just Exemption Forms   356

Chapter 12: Truth #9 - Unvaccinated Children Are Often Healthier Than Their Peers   373

Chapter 13: Truth #10 - People Who Say No to Vaccines Aren't Crazy—They're Paying Attention   392

Chapter 14: Now You Know   406

Preface

Back in 1988, while doing my undergraduate studies, I enrolled in an English class that would unknowingly alter the course of my life. The instructor gave us an assignment that would serve as our final exam: a research paper. We could choose any topic we wanted. She made it clear she wouldn't be grading us on *what* we wrote about, but *how* we wrote it: grammar, structure, organization. In other words, the mechanics of writing.

To most of my classmates, this assignment was just another box to check. But to me, it was something far more. It was my moment.

I felt like Ralphie in *A Christmas Story*, dreaming of the day he'd turn in his report on the Red Ryder Carbine Action 200-Shot Range Model Air Rifle and be showered in praise. That was me. But instead of a BB gun, I finally had the chance to write about something I had carried close to my heart since childhood… the vaccine dilemma.

You see, I had never received a single vaccine as a child. That always made me different, and I was proud of it. Whenever I asked my father why, he would just say, "They're not good for us. I'll explain one day." And I trusted him. But now I was in college, and the time had come to search for the truth myself. He encouraged me to take this opportunity to explore the issue deeply — and I did.

The assignment required us to cite our sources, so I began my search for evidence to support what I had always believed. But in 1988, that wasn't easy. Back then, almost all published literature echoed the same one-sided view — that vaccines were safe and essential. Still, I pressed on. During my search, I met a young married couple who shared my skepticism, so I interviewed them. They had a health philosophy which supported what they believed but, like me, hadn't read much on the subject yet. They had recently purchased a book that looked promising. They lent it to me with one simple request: highlight what I found important so they could focus on those parts when they eventually read it. I returned it with nearly the whole book highlighted.

That book opened my eyes and reinforced what I had felt intuitively for years. Along with a few other sources, it helped me craft a research paper that was heartfelt, well-structured, and — in my eyes — incredibly important. I turned it in on the second-to-last day of class, confident and excited. I believed it would finally answer the question people had asked me my whole life: *"Why weren't you vaccinated?"*

I was proud. It was my "Red Ryder" moment.

But at the final class, my excitement came crashing down. The instructor returned our papers, reminding us that the grade on this paper was our final grade for the course — and she had no time to discuss it before heading home to New York for Christmas. I looked down and saw a big, red **C-** on my paper. I was stunned.

Her comments in the margins weren't about grammar or sentence structure. They were full of outrage: "How can you say this?!" "What about polio?!" Clearly, she had graded me on content, not mechanics, and didn't agree with my position. I had followed the rules, cited my sources, and presented my case. But that didn't matter. I couldn't challenge her; she was already on a plane.

So I made an appointment with the head of the English department. He was gracious and understanding. He agreed that my grammar and writing were solid, and he acknowledged that my instructor should have graded me accordingly. But he wouldn't override her grade. What he did offer was something even more valuable: advice. He told me that the topic I had chosen was far too complex and important to be reduced to a small college research paper. "If you really want to take this on," he said, "do it justice. Take the time and effort it truly deserves."

That moment lit a fire in me. One that has never gone out.

For more than 35 years since, I have researched, studied, and examined vaccines from both sides of the debate. I've pored over scientific literature, historical records, manufacturer data, personal accounts, and public health reports. I've looked at what's said, and what's left unsaid.

This book is a result of that journey. It's the research paper I never got to write. The full version, the complete picture, the truth I've spent decades pursuing.

To that English teacher whose name I've long forgotten: thank you. You unknowingly fueled the passion that drives this work.

And to every parent, student, educator, healthcare professional, and truth-seeker reading this — may this book offer clarity, challenge assumptions, and inspire you to dig deeper. The truth is never afraid of questions. And when it comes to something as vital as the health and safety of future generations, we owe it to ourselves to ask the hard ones.

Introduction

You won't hear your doctor tell you about the information in this book. Why? Because they can't. It's not that they're ill-intentioned or lacking in compassion. It's because, for one reason or another, they simply don't know it—or they're afraid to share it. Afraid of the consequences. Afraid of being sanctioned. Afraid of losing their license. It happens. More often than you think. The truth gets buried, and potential whistleblowers are silenced before they can even speak. But I'm not afraid. I'm not bound by the same restrictions.

You see, I'm a Doctor of Chiropractic, and the AMA, the medical boards, they have no jurisdiction over me. I'm not dependent on their approval, and they can't take away my license. And I'm willing to speak.

Why? Because I've spent more than 35 years investigating, researching, studying, and teaching others about this topic. I've looked at both sides of the debate with a critical eye, and I've dug deep into the information that's hidden from the public. I've used my education about the body and it's amazing physiology to hone my ability to think critically, to question the status quo, and to draw conclusions based on truth—facts that many would prefer to keep hidden.

But this isn't just intellectual curiosity for me. This is personal. I know the devastating effects vaccinations can have on children and adults. I've seen the pain, the suffering, and the lives altered—forever. The reactions, the complications, the silent consequences that most people never hear about. And I can't stay quiet about it any longer. I can't let this truth remain buried, not when I know how many people are suffering in silence.

I'm also a test subject. I am living proof that it's possible to thrive without vaccinations. You see, I've never been vaccinated in my entire life—and yet here I am, not just surviving but thriving. Healthier than my peers, my friends, my classmates, my neighbors. While others have battled sickness after sickness, I've been largely untouched, a healthy anomaly.

When childhood illnesses came my way, my body fought them off naturally, swiftly, and without the need for medications. No antibiotics. No over-the-counter drugs. No vaccines. Just the natural strength of a body that knew how to heal itself. And now I enjoy lifelong immunity as the reward.

But it doesn't stop with me. None of my four siblings were vaccinated either. Not a single one. And guess what? We were all healthy. Healthier than most of the children around us. And it gets better. My children have never been vaccinated. They've grown into healthy, thriving adults—each of them surpassing their peers in terms of health and vitality.

And now, my nieces and nephews, those who chose the same path, are raising their own children—vaccination-free—and once again, the results speak for themselves. Dozens of us, all showing the same results, and the same lifelong immunity.

This is not just a personal story. It's not just a one-off anomaly. It's a living, breathing case study in thriving without vaccinations. But don't take my word for it. There are millions of people around the world who have made the choice to forgo vaccines for their children—and the results are undeniable.

So, what makes me qualified to write this book? I'm a doctor. I'm a researcher. I'm an author. But more than that, I am living proof. I am unvaccinated, and I am thriving. I am a part of a growing community of millions who have chosen a different path—and I have the results to show for it.

While educating others about vaccinations, I've always told them that my job isn't to convince them to vaccinate or not vaccinate. That's not my role. My job is to educate—to offer the whole picture, the information that's so often left out of the conversation—so that people can make truly informed decisions for themselves. Every one of us is responsible for our own health and the health of our children. That responsibility does not belong to me. It does not belong to your pediatrician. It does not belong to your family doctor, the AMA, the American Academy of Pediatrics, the CDC, or the pharmaceutical industry. It belongs to *you*. But in order to make good, responsible decisions, you need access to all the information—not just the sanitized version that those institutions hand out. That's what this book is designed to do. Not to make your choice for you. But to give you the *rest* of the story—so you can make a real, educated decision for your family.

Now, as you start reading this book, I want you to know that you'll no doubt hear certain common questions or comments that will attempt to challenge what you're learning. "What about polio?" "But vaccines save lives!" "Children need to be vaccinated to attend school!" These are the common refrains you will certainly encounter when you challenge the vaccine narrative. And when you do, you'll need more than just an opinion to respond. You'll need knowledge. You'll need data. You'll need certainty.

This book will give you all of that. It will give you the confidence to face these questions head-on, armed with the truth and the facts to back it up. It will provide you with the knowledge you need to engage in the vaccine debate on your own terms—and to stand firm in your own decisions, no matter what pressure you may face.

I commend you for having the courage to pick up this book and begin the process of understanding. I hope two things will happen as you go through these pages. First, I hope to open your eyes to information you have never been given before. Information that has been hidden, overlooked, or deliberately suppressed. Second, I hope you will open your mind to concepts that may be new to you, allowing you to grow your understanding and form your own conclusions. You will leave this book with a deeper, clearer perspective that will empower you to make informed decisions for yourself and your family.

So, as you turn the page, you're stepping into a world of discovery. A world where hidden truths are exposed, where conventional wisdom is challenged, and where critical thinking is encouraged. This book will not just present you with facts; it will empower you to think for yourself, to challenge the narratives you've been fed, and to make decisions that are in line with the truth, not with fear or blind obedience.

Welcome to the journey. The journey of discovering the Top 10 Truths About Vaccinations. This isn't just about vaccines—it's about understanding the larger systems at play, the way information is manipulated, and the way we can take back control over our own health. This journey could very well change everything you thought you knew about medicine, health, and the world we live in.

And remember, you are not alone.

Top 10 Truths About Vaccinations

1. **The Entire Vaccine Model Is Built on a Faulty Assumption**
   (Spoiler: It's not your immune system they trust—it's the needle.)
2. **Vaccines Don't Build Herd Immunity—They Undermine It**
   (Temporary protection ≠ lasting public health.)
3. **Vaccines Didn't Save Us from Disease—We Were Already Winning**
   (Mortality dropped long before the shots showed up.)
4. **The "Safe and Effective" Mantra Is a Marketing Line—Not Science**
   (Look closer. The studies don't say what you think they do.)
5. **Vaccines Can—and Do—Cause Serious Harm**
   (You won't hear this in a pediatrician's waiting room, but it's true.)
6. **There's Big Money Behind Every Shot**
   (When billions are on the line, safety becomes negotiable.)
7. **Your Doctor Is Supposed to Tell You More—They Usually Don't**
   (Informed consent isn't optional. It's the law.)
8. **Public School Does *Not* Require Vaccination—Just Exemption Forms**
   (They're hoping you won't look into it. You should.)
9. **Unvaccinated Children Are Often Healthier Than Their Peers**
   (The data is inconvenient—but it's there.)
10. **People Who Say No to Vaccines Aren't Crazy—They're Paying Attention**
    (They've read the fine print. You should too.)

Chapter 1: The Thinking Behind the Science

What if everything you thought you knew about health... wasn't entirely true?

What if the confidence you've placed in modern medicine, in its systems, its science, and its solutions, wasn't the result of careful critical thinking, but of inherited beliefs shaped by cultural momentum, authority, and repetition? What if your conclusions about vaccine safety, effectiveness, and necessity weren't *yours* at all, but the product of a way of thinking you've never consciously examined?

This book isn't just about vaccines. It's about how we *think* about vaccines, and health itself. And before we can even begin to weigh data, examine studies, or compare risks and benefits, we have to take a step back and ask a more foundational question: *What kind of thinking led us here in the first place?*

I know you probably didn't pick up this book hoping to dive into a conversation about philosophy or how we think, but stick with me for just a moment. The way we approach science (how we ask questions, interpret evidence, and form conclusions) isn't just background noise; it's the foundation for everything that follows.

This first chapter may not have the flashiest title, but it's the lens through which the rest of this book will come into focus. If we skip over the thinking behind the science, we risk missing the entire point of what the science is actually saying. So trust me, it's worth a few pages to understand *how* we think, before jumping into *what* we think.

Think of this book as a roadmap for making informed decision, and this chapter as the legend in the corner of the map. You know, that little box with all the symbols and keys that help you understand what you're looking at? That's what this chapter is designed to do. It gives you the tools to read the terrain ahead, so you're not just following someone else's route—you're choosing your own. When it comes to making important decisions about vaccinations, you deserve a clear path, not a blindfold.

Most people assume that science is an immovable monument to truth, that its conclusions are final and its authority unquestionable. But science is a process, not a belief system. And that process depends on the quality of thinking behind it.

That's where things get interesting. Because how we *think*—or the mental framework we bring to the table—shapes what we accept as truth. It determines whether we ask questions or swallow the answers whole.

So before we talk vaccines, before the stats, the studies, the scandals, we need to talk about something else first: *how we reason.*

I know. Thinking about *thinking* sounds like the fastest way to lose a reader. But hang with me. Because once you see how ideas are formed, how "facts" are framed, and how science is often built on assumptions... you'll never look at a medical recommendation the same way again.

Critical Decisions Require Critical Thinking

You've probably heard people say things like, "The science is settled," or "That doesn't prove anything." Statements like these aren't meant to spark discussion, they're meant to shut you down and shut you up. The goal is to stop you from asking questions. But if you look closer, they also reveal something deeper: the *reasoning style* behind them. These phrases reflect how the speaker is processing the world, and how they decide what counts as truth.

The two main styles are *inductive* and *deductive* reasoning. Knowing the difference isn't just academic. It's how you figure out whether someone is chasing the truth, or just defending their narrative.

So, before we talk about the shots, the science, or the statistics, let's take a step back and look at the mental tools we all use to make sense of them. Once we understand how reasoning works, we'll be in a much better place to talk about vaccines clearly, calmly, and thoughtfully.

Let's start with something simple. Say you walk past a neighbor's house every morning and always see a golden retriever in the yard. After a few weeks, you might think, "Those folks must own that dog."

That's *inductive reasoning*. You're going from repeated observations to a general conclusion. It seems reasonable. You've seen the pattern, so you assume the pattern explains the truth.

But not so fast. Maybe it's not their dog. Maybe it belongs to someone next door and just likes to hang out in that yard. Maybe the homeowners run a pet-sitting business. Or maybe the dog is a stray with impeccable taste in neighborhoods.

The point is, your conclusion is a guess. A good one, maybe— but still a guess. That's the limitation of induction: it's always *probable*, never guaranteed.

Now let's reinforce that idea with something a little messier. Imagine this:

You walk into your backyard and notice a pile of poop. And just like always, you see a cloud of flies buzzing around it.
So you think, "Ugh—those flies must've caused the poop."

That's inductive reasoning again. You saw two things happen together, so you assumed one caused the other. But just because two things show up together doesn't mean they're related in the way you think.

Now let's rewind and look at it deductively.

You know certain things to be absolutely true (premises), and from them you can draw an *accurate* conclusion.

> **Premise 1**: I have a dog.
> **Premise 2**: My dog uses the backyard to poop.
> **Premise 3**: Flies are attracted to poop.
> **Conclusion**: My dog made the poop, and that poop attracted the flies.

See the difference?

This is *deductive reasoning.* You start with known facts, apply them logically, and arrive at a conclusion that has to be true—as long as your premises are sound.

Induction says, "I keep seeing flies and poop together, so flies must cause poop."

Deduction says, "Poop attracts flies, and I have a dog, so the dog did it."

One is a guess built on repetition.

The other is a logical sequence built on principles.

And now you can probably see why this matters—not just for backyard hygiene, but for how we interpret science, medicine, and public health claims.

When people say, "When we vaccinate, we see fewer cases of disease," they're using inductive logic. They're seeing a pattern and forming a conclusion. But unless they test that pattern rigorously, ask what else might explain the trend, rule out other causes, and challenge their own assumptions, they could be getting it completely backwards.

Which brings us to the real issue: In medicine, sloppy reasoning doesn't just lead to dirty shoes, it leads to bad science, misdiagnosis, and harmful policy.

So again, before we dive into the science of vaccines, we have to sharpen the tools we're using to interpret that science.

Do we want to guess? Or do we want to know?

Think Like Sherlock

Imagine you're walking down Baker Street in London and find yourself inside the cozy, cluttered study of 221B, home to the world's most famous detective: Sherlock Holmes.*

A client bursts through the door, frantic… a priceless family heirloom has gone missing. The local police have already formed their theory: "It must have been the housemaid, she was the only one near the room at the time!" They're using *inductive reasoning*. They saw that she was nearby, and from that single observation, they're building a theory, and then jumped to a general conclusion based on a specific clue.

But Holmes? Holmes doesn't rush to conclusions. He leans back in his armchair, steeples his fingers, and begins his work using *deductive reasoning*.

> *"You see, Watson,"* he says coolly, *"It is a capital mistake to theorize before one has data. Insensibly, one begins to twist facts to suit theories, instead of theories to suit facts."**

*Sir Arthur Conan Doyle, A Scandal in Bohemia, 1891.

Holmes starts not with the observation, but with the *principles* of logic, human behavior, and physical evidence. He forms a hypothesis based on what should logically be true *if* the theory is correct—then tests that theory by seeking out specific evidence.

Premise 1: If the maid stole the heirloom, her fingerprints would be on the inside of the locked drawer.
Premise 2: The drawer was locked, and the key was kept in a hidden compartment.
Observation: The drawer was pried open, and no fingerprints are present — but there is a boot print that matches a man's boot.

"Elementary," Holmes declares. "The maid is innocent. The window was forced open, and the mud from the garden proves the thief entered from outside. The boot print, the broken latch, and the absence of fingerprints — all consistent with *my original theory*, and inconsistent with the police's."*

He didn't start with what he saw and build a theory (*inductive reasoning*). He started with a broad principle — "If X is true, then Y must be observed." And when Y wasn't observed, he eliminated X.

Why Deduction Wins (Especially in Critical Thinking)

Holmes shows us the power of deduction:

Deductive reasoning filters out falsehoods. It's not swayed by coincidence or correlation. Just because someone is nearby doesn't mean they're guilty.

It's testable. Holmes's hypotheses must align with *all* observed facts, or they're discarded.

It gets to the root of the truth, instead of stopping at the surface.

While inductive reasoning can help us explore new ideas and detect patterns, it's often vulnerable to error — especially when the stakes are high and the facts must be exact.

Deductive reasoning, on the other hand, like Sherlock Holmes's method, is about testing theories with precision, weeding out errors, and following logic to the truth.

In science, health, law, and life, we'd all do well to ask: *Am I thinking like the police… or like Holmes?*

Health: A Matter of Perspective

Now, let's shift gears—but not really. Because how we think about *reasoning* is directly tied to how we think about *health*.

Think about it: if your mindset is to attack anything that looks like disease, you're going to see the body as a battlefield. Germs are the enemy. Doctors are soldiers. And treatments are weapons. That's the *Pathogenic Model* of health. The one most people know. It defines health by the absence of disease, and sees healing as a war against whatever's invading the system.

Like our backyard example. The pathogenic model's solution would be to use bug spray and fly traps to kill the flies, hoping the poop would go away.

But there's another way to think about it.

It's called the *Salutogenic Model,* and it asks different questions:

Not "What caused the illness?" But "What supports health?"

This model doesn't just look at what went wrong. It studies what makes people resilient in the face of stress, infection, trauma, or even aging. It values strength, adaptability, and vitality, not just the absence of symptoms.

So while the pathogenic model asks how to kill the germ, the salutogenic model asks how to resist it *before* it becomes a problem. It asks "how do we strengthen the host?"

Think about how differently these two mindsets approach vaccines.

In the pathogenic model, vaccines are tools, preemptive strikes to eliminate threats.

In the salutogenic model, you also have to ask:

Does this intervention support the body's long-term health? Does it build resilience, or just suppress symptoms?

Most people never think about health this way. They've been trained to equate "not sick" with "healthy." But health is more than a lack of disease, it's the presence of well-being.

Even the World Health Organization admits this. They have adopted Dorland's Medical Dictionary's definition of health:

"Health: A state of optimal physical, mental, and social well-being, *not merely the absence of disease or infirmity.*"
– Dorland's Medical Dictionary

So before we examine vaccines—what they are, what they do, and what they claim—we need to be crystal clear about the lens we're using. Because if two people define "health" differently, they're not just disagreeing, they're speaking different languages.

Are you ready? Because now that we've sharpened our thinking skills and adjusted our lenses, we can begin.

Let's talk about the Top 10 Truths About Vaccinations.

Chapter 2: Truth #1 - The Entire Vaccine Model Is Built on a Faulty Assumption

(Spoiler: It's not your immune system they trust—it's the needle.)

The entire practice of vaccination rests on a single belief: *that specific germs cause specific diseases*, and therefore if you can train the body to recognize and fight those germs before they cause harm, you can prevent illness altogether.

This belief is the one that Modern Medicine has adopted and trained us to follow. It's called the Germ Theory of Disease.

The Germ Theory

The germ theory proposes that microorganisms, things like bacteria, viruses, and other tiny pathogens, are the primary cause of infectious diseases. Before this theory, people wondered why diseases spread or how to stop them. There were many scientists, doctors, chemists, and thinkers during those days who were trying to discover the cause for all disease.

One scientist, *Louis Pasteur* theorized that germs were the culprits behind illnesses, which led to his next question: *Can we stop these invaders before they do damage?*

He aligned with the pathogenic model, and that's where the vaccination steam engine really started to roll.

Vaccines are thought to be a *preemptive strike,* based on the germ theory. Without the germ theory, vaccination as we know it wouldn't exist.

At first glance, the idea may seem clear-cut: *germs cause disease*. Most of us grew up hearing that message—wash your hands, cover your mouth, avoid sick people. All of this was based on the belief that tiny, invisible microbes are responsible for making us sick.

However, what we now refer to as the *Germ Theory of Disease* remains just that… a *theory*. But what does it mean for something to be a theory? A theory is essentially… a belief.

The belief that germs cause disease marked a radical shift in society's understanding of health. While the germ theory remains a framework rather than an absolute fact, it has undeniably transformed modern medicine and shaped a substantial portion of society's faith in medical practices. But why has this theory garnered such widespread acceptance?

One compelling reason lies in its alignment with the classic "Hero vs. Villain" narrative. Humanity has an inherent desire to frame our struggles in terms of clear dichotomies—identifying heroes who can rescue us from villains. In a time of desperation, when people fell ill for mysterious reasons and sought guidance, the search for solutions created fertile ground for this narrative.

Pasteur, a prominent figure, speaker, and influencer of the time, effectively crafted a classic storyline. In this narrative, germs emerged as the villain—unseen, insidious agents responsible for illness and suffering. On the other hand, the hero in this tale was not merely medical practitioners or hospitals but rather the development and use of drugs and vaccines aimed at combating these microbial foes.

The discovery of microscopic organisms, and the idea that they could actually invade the body and cause harm, changed everything. It gave medicine a new villain: *the pathogen.*

The germ theory helped launch weapons like antibiotics, vaccines, sterilization techniques, and much of what most people now consider to be basic healthcare. But like all powerful ideas, it also came with some pretty lofty assumptions—especially the idea that if we can just kill the germs, we can eliminate all disease. That assumption narrowed our focus. It placed the microbe at the center of the conversation, and pushed the host (the human body and its own ability to stay healthy) into the background.

Understanding the germ theory's history and its influence on modern medicine is key, not just for grasping how we fight disease today, but for asking bigger questions about what causes illness in the first place. Over a century and a half after Louis Pasteur formulated the germ theory, one must ask: have we truly achieved the eradication of disease?

In this chapter, I will delve into the origins of the germ theory, tracing its development, and examine the opposing viewpoints that exist, despite being less widely promoted.

Additionally, I will present evidence demonstrating how the germ theory can be challenged based on factual information, logical reasoning, and even its own supporting framework.

How the Germ Theory of Disease Came to Be

It might appear as obvious to us today to say that germs cause disease, but that idea is actually pretty new in the grand timeline of medicine.

For thousands of years, people had all sorts of other explanations for where they thought illness came from – including bad air, evil spirits, or imbalances in the body's fluids. Nobody had ever seen a microbe, let alone suspected one could make you sick.

The story of the Germ Theory of Disease really starts to take shape in the 1600s, when a Dutch fabric merchant named *Antonie van Leeuwenhoek* started tinkering with microscopes. He wasn't a doctor or scientist in the traditional sense, but he had a curious mind. When he looked at water through his handmade lenses, he saw a whole world of, what he called, tiny "animalcules"—what we now know as microorganisms. He didn't know what they were doing in there, but he proved they existed.

Fast forward to the 1800s, and we start seeing some advancements in the discovery of microorganisms. In Italy, *Agostino Bassi* showed that a fungus was causing disease in silkworms. Around the same time, *Ignaz Semmelweis*, a Hungarian doctor, made a shocking discovery: when doctors washed their hands, fewer women died during childbirth.

Then came Louis Pasteur, who was a French chemist, and he changed everything. In the mid-1800s, he proved that microbes were doing specific things, like causing food to spoil or wine to turn sour. Then he took it further and showed that microbes could be passed between people and animals.

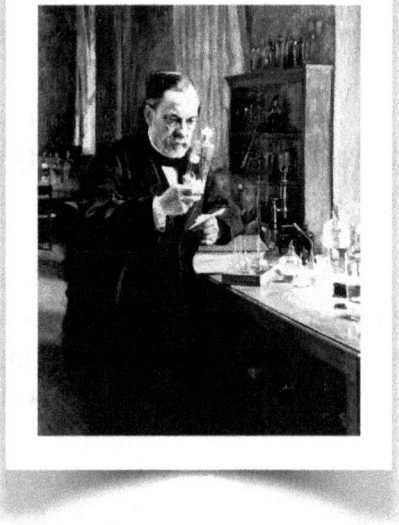

Pasteur then developed early vaccines for diseases like anthrax and rabies, and because he was so politically connected and had a talent for public communication and securing institutional support, he convinced people that germs were real, *and they were dangerous*.

Why are germs even here?

We're used to thinking of bacteria and viruses as enemies, invaders that sneak into the body and make us sick. But there's another perspective that flips that idea on its head: what if microbes aren't so much the *cause* of disease, but the *cleanup crew* that shows up after something has already gone wrong?

You see, bacteria and viruses play a natural, biological role on our planet. Their job is to *break down dead or dying organic material.*

Just like how microbes cause a dead tree in the forest to decay, they also decompose any organic tissue that is no longer healthy. They thrive in areas where the body's internal environment has become weak, acidic, toxic, or otherwise imbalanced.

This doesn't mean that we should ignore them (like in cases of sanitation, surgery, or childbirth, etc.), but it does suggest a shift in focus. Instead of asking, *"What germ caused this disease?"*, we might ask, *"What made the tissue vulnerable in the first place?"* Or, *"Why did the environment inside the body become one where these microbes could thrive?"*

In this framework, bacteria don't attack healthy cells. They colonize in tissues that are already damaged or inflamed. And viruses, which aren't alive in the traditional sense, may act more like messengers or triggers for cellular cleanup, not assassins targeting the body without reason.

So rather than being the villains of the story, bacteria and viruses could be seen more like *first responders*, arriving on the scene of a *biological breakdown*. Their presence may signal that a deeper problem already exists, and that the body's *terrain* needs internal support, not external defense.

This doesn't erase the role microbes can play in illness. But it does invite a broader perspective: one where health is not about avoiding germs, but about creating an internal environment where disease can't take hold in the first place.

Have you ever thought about what would happen if bacteria didn't exist?

It's a little weird to imagine, but without bacteria, we'd be in big trouble. In fact, the world would be covered in dead things. Dead animals, plants, food… just piling up with nowhere to go. Why? Again, because bacteria's job in nature is to break down dead and dying tissue. That's their purpose. That's why they're here.

Think about that fallen tree in the forest. Over time, it starts to rot and break apart. That's not just nature "doing its thing", that's bacteria and other microbes going to work, breaking down the wood, bark, and leaves into soil and nutrients. Bacteria are recycling machines!

The same thing happens when an animal dies. Bacteria move in and start the clean-up process, breaking down the body so it can return to the earth.

Imagine you leave a piece of raw chicken out on the kitchen counter overnight. You forget it's there. The next morning, it smells awful. It's slimy. Maybe even discolored. What happened? *Bacteria happened.*

When that meat sat out, bacteria in the environment (ones already on the surface of the chicken or floating through the air) got to work. To them, that chicken is no longer living tissue; it's a free buffet. Their job? *To break it down.* And they're very good at it. In fact, the smell and sliminess are signs that they're doing exactly what they're supposed to do: decomposing something that's dead.

The same thing goes for your fruit bowl. Leave a banana or a tomato out too long and it gets soft, mushy, and eventually moldy. That's not just the fruit "going bad" on its own. It's bacteria and other microorganisms breaking down that dying produce into simpler organic matter. Left long enough, it'll rot all the way down to sludge and juice.

Why does this matter? Because it shows that bacteria's natural role is cleanup. They don't just show up to make things gross, they show up to recycle dead things and return them to the environment. In nature, it's brilliant. Without bacteria, fallen trees wouldn't rot, dead animals wouldn't decompose, and old food wouldn't break down. The world would be one big pile of dead stuff. Not exactly a livable planet.

So when you see food spoil, you're not just seeing decay, you're seeing bacteria doing their job.

And remember: they don't only do this outside your body. The same kind of bacteria that break down old produce are related to the bacteria in your gut that help break down food after you eat it. Whether it's a rotting apple on the counter or a salad in your stomach, bacteria know what to do: break it down, reuse it, and keep the cycle of life moving.

You can think of it like this: the food you eat is kind of like "dead material" by the time it hits your stomach and intestines. The gut bacteria come in and break it down further, helping you absorb nutrients and keeping your digestion running smoothly. It's a partnership.

So, whether it's decomposing a fallen log in the forest or breaking down your lunch after a sandwich, bacteria are nature's clean-up crew. Their role isn't to harm, it's to transform, recycle, and support life.

By the late 1800s, the germ theory had gone from a radical idea to the foundation of modern medicine. While Louis Pasteur was busy developing his germ theory of disease, there was another scientist working on a very different idea: *Antoine Béchamp*. These two weren't exactly friendly collaborators. In fact, they were rivals. Both respected scientists in 19th-century France, but with very different views on what really causes disease.

Two Competing Views

Opposing Pasteur's "germs cause disease" idea, Antoine Béchamp formulated the *Terrain Theory* (sometimes called the H*ost Theory*). According to him, it's not the germs that matter most, it's the condition of your body's internal environment, or what he called the "terrain."

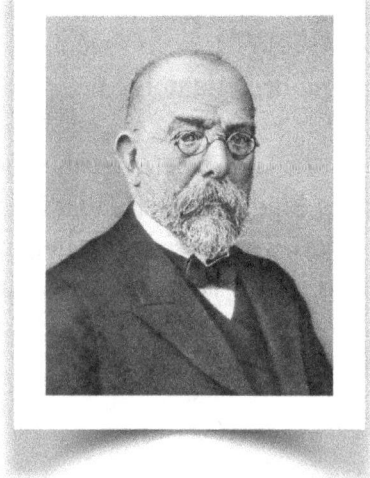

In his view, microbes don't *cause* disease. Instead, they show up because the body is already in a weakened, imbalanced, or unhealthy state. Basically, if your terrain is healthy, germs cannot thrive.

Think of the terrain theory as analogous to the growth of a seed. If you place that seed in a box of sand, neglect to water it, and keep it in a completely dark room, it will remain dormant and will not sprout into a plant. However, if you take the same seed and plant it in nutrient-rich potting soil, provide adequate water, fertilize it, and position it where it can receive sunlight, that seed will not only sprout but will thrive and grow into a healthy plant.

The same principle applies to the terrain theory in relation to health. If bacteria or viruses enter an environment that is inhospitable to their survival, such as a healthy body with robust tissues, they will struggle to establish a foothold. They won't be able to replicate and cause harm.

In contrast, if these microbes find a suitable terrain in which to thrive, such as an unhealthy body or weakened tissues, they will proliferate and potentially result in destructive consequences (disease).

It is important to remember that the purpose of germs in nature is to break down dead, dying, or weakened tissue. They do not discriminate; they simply fulfill their biological role within the ecosystem.

Therefore it is the "soil", or the overall health of the body, that ultimately determines the outcome. This emphasizes the importance of maintaining a healthy internal environment rather than on the eradication of germs.

Not Just a Scientific Disagreement

Béchamp was the older of the two. He was a well respected scientist and had deep roots in biological chemistry. Pasteur, meanwhile, was very skilled in the political and public spheres. He had a knack for winning support from institutions and the public, and he communicated his ideas in a way that really caught on.

Their rivalry wasn't just about science, it got personal. They clashed publicly and often. And in the end, it was Pasteur who gained more fame, official backing, and a lasting place in history books.

Louis Pasteur
Germ Theory of Disease

Aspect	Description
Core Idea	Microorganisms (germs) from the outside invade the body and cause disease.
Cause of Disease	Specific external pathogens.
Focus of Treatment	Kill or eliminate the pathogen (e.g., with antibiotics, vaccines, sterilization).
View of the Body	A mostly passive host that becomes sick when invaded by germs.
Prevention Strategy	Avoid or destroy pathogens before they can infect (e.g., vaccination, hygiene).

Legacy	Foundation for modern Western medicine, vaccines, and public health policies. Main principle of the Pathogenic Model of healthcare.

Antoine Béchamp
Terrain (Host) Theory of Disease

Aspect	Description
Core Idea	Disease arises when the body's internal environment (terrain) is unhealthy.
Cause of Disease	A weakened or toxic internal environment that allows microbes to become harmful.
Focus of Treatment	Strengthen and support the body's natural healing systems.
View of the Body	An active participant in health; germs only thrive in unhealthy conditions.
Prevention Strategy	Keep the body healthy and in balance so that disease doesn't take hold.
Legacy	Less accepted by mainstream medicine, but influential in holistic, wellness, and salutogenic practices.

Pasteur saw germs as the enemy to be eradicated. He used inductive reasoning. He started with several small observations: *whenever there was disease, there were microorganisms*. From there he developed a large conclusion: *germs cause disease*.

Béchamp saw a weakened body as the real problem, and germs as opportunists. He used deductive reasoning. He started with an accurate premise: T*he role of germs is to break down dead, dying, or weakened tissue.* His conclusions were small and accurate: *if the body becomes weakened, then germs will begin their natural process and break it down, thus causing illness.* It's the "soil", not the "seed".

Koch's Postulates

Not long after Pasteur formulated his germ theory, a German doctor named *Robert Koch* (pronounced "Coke") was trying to figure out some things he deemed necessary: *How can we prove the germ theory, and how do we know if a specific germ actually causes a specific disease?*

During this period, early scientists were striving to understand the tiny, invisible organisms we now identify as bacteria and viruses, and whether they could truly be responsible for causing illness in humans. This idea was relatively novel at the time. To address this uncertainty, Robert Koch formulated a set of four steps—similar to a checklist—to prove whether a specific germ was indeed the primary cause of a disease. These steps are known as *Koch's Postulates*. Let me walk you through them:

Koch's 4 Postulates:

1. **The microorganisms must be found in abundance of *every* case of the disease, but cannot be found in healthy cases.**

So if a host animal has a disease, Koch said you should always be able to find the suspected pathogen in them. If someone *doesn't* have the disease, they *cannot* have that pathogen.

2. **You have to be able to isolate the germ from the sick host and grow it in a lab.**
Basically, take the germ out of the sick host and grow it on its own, in a petri dish or something like that, so you know you're only dealing with *that* specific germ.

3. **When you introduce the germ into a healthy subject, it must cause the same disease.**
In other words, if you give the bacteria from that petri dish, to a healthy lab animal, that new animal should get sick in the same way as the original animal did.

4. **You have to be able to re-isolate the same germ from the newly sick host.**
After that healthy subject gets sick, you should be able to take the bacteria out again and prove it's the *same* one you started with.

Seems pretty logical, right? Koch's Postulates seemed to help make the case that certain microbes were behind specific diseases. It gave scientists a step-by-step method to prove what was causing illness.

Or did it?!

Here's the thing... Koch's Postulates were actually meant to *prove* the germ theory. Ironically, they end up poking some pretty big holes in it.

Allow me to explain. Koch's *first postulate* says this: A disease-causing organism must be found in abundance in every case of the disease—*and not found in healthy individuals.*

Sounds pretty straightforward, right? If you're sick with a particular disease, the microbe causing it should be present. However, according to Koch's first postulate, if you're healthy, *it shouldn't be.* This postulate was meant to create a clear cause-and-effect relationship between a germ and a disease.

But here's the kicker: in real life, this doesn't always hold true. In fact, there are *many* cases where people are exposed to a so-called "pathogen," and yet never develop the disease. In other words, healthy people can still have the germ... and not be sick. Let's look at a few well-known examples:

HIV/AIDS

Plenty of people test HIV-positive but never go on to develop AIDS. Some remain completely healthy for years, even decades. So... if HIV is the pathogen, why don't they all get sick?

COVID-19

Remember the wave of testing during the Covid pandemic? Tons of people tested positive for the virus but never had a single symptom. During this time, we were told there were different possible outcomes if you tested positive for the virus:

- You might get severely ill,
- You might just have a mild cold,
- Or… you might feel totally fine.

That last group (people who never got sick at all) *totally contradicts Koch's first postulate*. If the virus is the cause, why didn't everyone show symptoms?

Herpes Simplex Virus 1 (HSV-1)

This virus is known for causing cold sores, but many people who carry the virus never get one. Romantic couples kiss regularly. In many cases even though one partner gets cold sores, the other never does despite repeated exposure.

Hepatitis C

Here's another one: hepatitis C is often called a "silent disease" because so many people have no symptoms at all. In fact, around half the people with hepatitis C don't even know they have it. Again, the virus is present, but the disease isn't.

And what's the explanation for all these contradictions?

You've probably heard the term *"asymptomatic carrier"*. This term is the medical community's way of backing out of the corner they've painted themselves into by saying, "Okay, this person has the pathogen... and for some reason, they're just not sick, so we'll give a label—asymptomatic carrier". It's a label that's now used frequently.

However if you think about it, it kind of admits the problem. Because once you allow for the idea that someone can carry a pathogen and *not* develop disease, you've essentially *violated Koch's first postulate*. You're saying the germ alone doesn't necessarily cause illness—it depends on the person, their immune system, or something else entirely.

So here's the bottom line: While Koch's Postulates were meant to support the germ theory of disease, examples like these show us the opposite... that the host's condition, or their internal environment, matters much more, than the germ itself.

Here's a thought-provoking scenario: Doctors around the globe see sick patients in their offices on a daily basis. These individuals, seeking care for their illnesses, often share the same room, sitting knee to knee with the healthcare practitioner during examinations.

Commands like "Stick out your tongue and say 'Ahhh'" are

> "If the 'germ theory of disease' were correct, there'd be no one living to believe it"
> -Dr. B.J. Palmer

commonplace, requiring doctors to lean in closely to inspect the back of the patient's throat, all while the patient breathes near the examiner.

If germs truly caused disease as the primary explanation, one might wonder: wouldn't every doctor fall ill every day? Would there be any doctors left to care for patients if exposure to germs invariably resulted in sickness, disease, or death?

This scenario invites reflection on the relative health and resilience of healthcare providers in these environments. Despite their frequent contact with sick individuals, many doctors remain healthy.

This observation raises important questions about the role of the immune system, overall health, and the potential influence of the environment on susceptibility to illness.

And, if those examples are not enough to emphasize that germs don't cause disease, let's take a moment to look at one of the most fascinating (and rarely discussed) cases in medical history: the Soviet conjoined twins *Masha and Dasha Krivoshlyapova.*

Masha and Dasha

Born in 1950, these twins were physically connected in a truly unique way. Each had her own head, brain, and spinal cord. Each had one arm, and they shared two legs. They also had two separate immune systems—but, critically, they shared the same bloodstream.[4]

Now think about that: two immune systems, one circulatory system. This means any pathogen (a virus, bacteria, etc.) that entered one sister's blood would almost instantly be shared with the other. In theory, based on the germ theory of disease, both girls should get sick at the same time, in the same way. After all, they were literally sharing the same infected blood.

But that's not what happened.

Time and again, doctors observed that one sister would come down with a fever, or a cold, or an infection, while the other remained completely fine.[4] Same blood. Same pathogen. Totally different outcomes.

This strange case throws a serious wrench into one of the oldest foundations of infectious disease theory: *Koch's Postulates.* Remember, his first postulate is this:

"The microorganism must be found in all organisms suffering from the disease, but not in healthy organisms."[3]

In other words, if you're sick, you have the germ; and if you're healthy, you don't. But Masha and Dasha challenge that idea head-on. In their case, the germ was clearly present in both sisters' blood, but *only one of them would get sick.*

According to Koch's logic, that simply shouldn't happen.

This case doesn't just stretch the limits of Germ Theory, it cracks it wide open. It suggests that germs alone don't make us sick. Instead, it points to a bigger picture, one where the state of the host's immune system, internal environment, stress levels, and more determine whether or not an illness actually takes hold.[1,2]

In fact, this is exactly what many researchers and health thinkers argue today: that the terrain (the condition of the body) matters more than the germ. The presence of bacteria or viruses in the body doesn't necessarily equal disease. It's how the body handles that microbe that makes all the difference.

So while the story of Masha and Dasha may not be widely known, it's one of the most compelling real-life examples that show why we need to rethink what really causes illness, and question whether the germ theory, at least in its original, rigid form, is the full story.

Louis Pasteur and Robert Koch observed patterns and gathered evidence over time to make generalizations about the relationship between microorganisms and disease. They primarily used inductive reasoning to formulate their conclusions.

Antoine Béchamp however, noticed that diseases were more likely to develop in bodies that were out of balance, either due to poor nutrition, toxins, or other stressors. From these observations, he could then deduce that pathogens didn't directly cause disease on their own, but rather, their harmful effects were largely determined by the state of the host's body. He also emphasized that microorganisms were part of the body's natural ecosystem, and in a healthy body, they didn't cause harm.

Once Béchamp had established the *general principle* that the internal condition of the host is critical for disease development (and that pathogens themselves aren't the direct cause), he used deductive reasoning to apply this theory to specific situations. For example, once he concluded that an unhealthy host is more vulnerable, he could deduce that a person in poor health would be more likely to develop disease when exposed to a pathogen, even if others exposed to the same pathogen did not get sick.

After everything we've explored—from the foundational principles of inductive vs. deductive reasoning, to Koch's Postulates, to the case of Masha and Dasha, it becomes increasingly difficult to ignore the gaping holes in the germ theory of disease. While the germ theory has played a major historical role in shaping modern medicine, it largely rests on the premise that the microbe alone is to blame. But that's a bit like blaming the flies for the feces. Microbes may show up in disease, but they don't explain *why* one person gets sick and another doesn't, especially when two people literally share the same bloodstream, like Masha and Dasha, and only one shows symptoms.

Deductive reasoning forces us to ask better questions: If germs are the sole cause of illness, why isn't the outcome always the same when exposure occurs? Why are some people completely unaffected by pathogens that are supposedly deadly? These questions aren't fringe, they're logical, and they demand answers that germ theory cannot comfortably give.

That's where the terrain theory steps in, not as a rejection of microbes, but as a broader, more holistic lens. It says: focus on the soil, not just the seed. Strengthen the internal environment, our terrain, and the body becomes far less hospitable to disease, regardless of what germs are around. Louis Pasteur himself, toward the end of his life, reportedly admitted, *"The microbe is nothing. The terrain is everything."*[5] He spent a lifetime advancing the germ theory, but in the end, even he realized the truth lies deeper.

When we follow the evidence with deductive clarity, we don't just land on a better theory, we arrive at a better understanding of what it means to be truly healthy. And that, in the end, is what this conversation has been about: seeing beyond the microscope, and instead looking within.

So let's get this straight, if the entire premise of vaccination hinges on the germ theory, and the germ theory doesn't hold water, then the whole vaccination program isn't built on science, it's built on a house of cards.

Do we even need to keep going? Probably not. But we will.

Because once you see the cracks in the foundation, it's only fair to show you how deep they run.

Chapter Sources

1. Bechamp, A. (1911). The Blood and Its Third Anatomical Element. Philadelphia, PA: Boericke & Tafel.
2. Engel, G. L. (1977). The need for a new medical model: A challenge for biomedicine. *Science*, 196(4286), 129–136.
3. Koch, R. (1987). Classic papers in genetics: The etiology of tuberculosis (translation of 1890 publication). Garland Publishing.
4. Ryan, F. (1988). *The Forgotten Twins: Masha and Dasha*. BBC Horizon documentary transcript and commentary. (Available via archive sources and secondary literature)
5. Hume, E. (1989). Bechamp or Pasteur? A lost chapter in the history of biology. New Canaan, CT: Health Research.

Chapter 3: Immunology 101

Now that we understand that the principle upon which vaccination is based upon (the germ theory) is flawed, let us turn our attention to the fundamentals of vaccinations through the lens of basic immunology.

This foundational knowledge is covered in every medical school, chiropractic college, osteopathic school, and many institutions of higher education. Understanding the core principles of human immunology is critical, as it applies to vaccination in fundamental and significant ways.

Four Types of Immunity

The human body is a marvel of biological engineering, with its immune system serving as a sophisticated defense mechanism against a constant barrage of potential invaders. The complexity of this intricate network, composed of various cells, tissues, and signaling molecules, demonstrates how our bodies adapt to a diverse range of threats.

Despite the advanced nature of our immune responses, they are distilled into four primary types of immunity:

1. **Natural Active Immunity**
2. **Natural Passive Immunity**
3. **Artificial Active Immunity**
4. **Artificial Passive Immunity**

Each type plays a unique role in how our bodies recognize and combat infections, reflecting a delicate balance between innate defense strategies and acquired responses. In understanding these four categories, we gain valuable insight into the dynamic nature of our immune system and how it equips us to thrive in an ever-changing environment. This exploration into the different forms of immunity not only enhances our appreciation of human biology and physiology, it also informs our approaches to immunization and disease prevention.

Let's discuss each one.

Natural Active Immunity

Natural Active Immunity is acquired when the body is exposed to an antigen (germ) through natural means, enabling it to successfully defend itself against the invader. This response not only neutralizes the threat but also establishes a lifelong immunity to that specific antigen.

Whenever we encounter an external invader, be it bacteria, virus, or other microbe, our body responds swiftly, much like a local fire department rushing to extinguish a four-alarm blaze. This immediate and decisive action underscores the remarkable efficiency of our immune system.

The design of the human body is nothing short of extraordinary. We are not meant to live in constant fear of unseen attackers, cowering in anticipation of their next assault. Instead, we are designed to cohabitate harmoniously with all forms of life, including the myriad of microbes that share our environment. Our immune system exemplifies this concept through the cultivation of *Natural Active Immunity*, demonstrating our inherent ability to adapt and thrive in the face of pathogenic challenges.

Nowhere is this principle more apparent than in the fortification of the body, which consists of multiple layers of defense designed to protect us from external threats.

Picture a well-constructed fortress, like a fort or castle, equipped with several barriers that invaders must penetrate before even attempting to access its precious interior. Historically, these fortifications were often situated on cliffs or near bodies of water, serving as the first line of defense. A surrounding moat acted as a deterrent, slowing down unwelcome intruders attempting to reach the drawbridge. Tall walls, crafted from logs with spiked tops or sturdy stone blocks, provided an additional layer of security. Lookout towers manned by vigilant sentries kept watch day and night, ready to summon armed soldiers at a moment's notice if an enemy was detected. Various weapons of war, from bows and arrows to cannons and firearms, further bolstered defenses, safeguarding the families within.

Much like these historical fortifications, our bodies are designed with *several layers of defense* to fend off potential external invaders. Each component of the immune system works in harmony, mirroring the strategic architecture of a fortress, ensuring our safety and well-being in an often hostile environment.

These layers of defense include: skin, hair, mucus, excretion, expulsion, temperature, pH, white blood cells, antibodies, lymphatics, etc. Let's go through them in detail.

Layers of Defense

SKIN

Let's talk about something you probably don't think about much, your skin. It's easy to take it for granted because it's always there, covering every inch of your body. But believe it or not, your skin is actually your *first and most important line of defense* when it comes to protecting you from illness and infection.

Think of it as your body's natural armor, but way more advanced.

First off, your skin forms a *physical barrier* between your internal body and the outside world. It keeps out all kinds of potential invaders: bacteria, viruses, fungi, pollutants, you name it. Without this layer, your insides would be completely exposed and vulnerable.

And it's not just a single, flat sheet. Your skin is made up of *multiple layers*, the epidermis, dermis, and hypodermis, each with its own role in keeping you safe.

Now let's talk about what makes skin so unique. It's not stiff or hard like armor, but it's still strong and resilient. It can stretch, bend, and move with you, thanks to its elasticity and pliability. It protects you while still allowing you full freedom of motion.

Plus, skin isn't smooth and slick like glass. It has texture, with tiny ridges, pores, and hair follicles, all of which help it do its job.

Your skin plays a huge role in regulating body temperature. When you're hot, your sweat glands kick in to release moisture and cool you off. When you're cold, tiny muscles in your skin make your hair stand up (hello, goosebumps!) to help trap heat. It's part of your body's own built-in thermostat.

And let's not forget one of skin's coolest features: feeling. Your skin is loaded with nerve endings, allowing you to feel pain, pleasure, pressure, temperature, and touch. It helps you respond to your environment and avoid danger, like pulling your hand away from a hot stove or feeling something sharp before it cuts you, letting microbes in.

On top of the physical protection, your skin also acts as a *chemical defense*. It produces natural oils and sweat that create a slightly acidic environment, which makes it harder for harmful microbes to grow. It's like your skin has its own mini chemical warfare system.

And by the way, your skin is actually covered in bacteria—right now. Sounds gross, right? But don't worry, that's completely normal. In fact, many of these bacteria are your body's friends, not foes. One of the most common of these "friendly" microbes is *Staphylococcus aureus*, or commonly called *staph* for short.

Most of the time, *staph* just hangs out on your skin, minding its own business. It lives there symbiotically, meaning it gets a nice place to live, and in return, it helps keep other microbes in check. It's part of your body's natural ecosystem, what we call the skin microbiome. Your immune system recognizes it and usually lets it be, because it's not causing any harm.

Every now and then, though, *staph* can become a problem. It's kind of like a neighbor who's usually quiet but can cause serious trouble under the wrong circumstances.

When *staph* gets through the outer layers, caught in pores, or goes unchecked by your body, it can cause infections ranging from mild (like pimples or boils) to very serious—like *necrotizing fasciitis*, the scary condition most people know as *"flesh-eating bacteria"*.

The takeaway is that context matters. *Staph aureus* isn't inherently bad—it lives on us all the time without causing any problems. It only becomes dangerous when it gets into places it shouldn't be, or when your body isn't strong enough to keep it under control *(Terrain Theory, Chapter 2)*.

The skin microbiome is also another example which disproves the germ theory through Koch's Postulates. Let's quickly review:

As I previously stated, *Staph aureus* is routinely found on healthy skin. You could test a group of perfectly healthy people and easily find this bacteria on many of them. They're not sick, they're not showing any symptoms, and there's no disease in sight.

Yet, in other people, sometimes even the same strain of *Staph aureus* can cause devastating infections like *necrotizing fasciitis*. So, same bacteria… two completely different outcomes.

That directly contradicts Koch's first postulate. If the germ is present in healthy people and they're not sick, then it can't be said to *always* cause the disease. That breaks the neat cause-and-effect model of the germ theory, which the vaccine premise is based on. (Chapter 2)

Enter the Terrain Theory. Now here's where Antoine Béchamp's Terrain Theory comes in—and starts to make a lot more sense.

Béchamp argued that it's not the germ itself that causes disease, but the condition of the host—that is your body, your internal "terrain."

According to this view, bacteria like *Staph aureus* are opportunists. They live peacefully on healthy tissue, but when the terrain becomes compromised—due to a wound, a weak immune system, poor nutrition, stress, or other imbalances—the same bacteria can suddenly become harmful.

In other words, the state of your body determines the outcome, not just the presence of the germ.

Your skin, once again, plays a crucial role by keeping that boundary sealed. Penetrate the skin, and you open the door for disaster.

HAIR

We usually think of hair in terms of style, grooming, or maybe the nuisance of plucking and shaving. But did you know that hair actually plays a large role in your immune defense system? Yep. Those tiny strands all over your body aren't just for looks. They're part of your built-in, frontline security system, working quietly to keep invaders out and protect your inner terrain.

Let's start with the hair you see on your arms, legs, and other parts of your body. While it might seem like it's just there for warmth or appearance, it actually acts like an early warning sensor. Hair on the skin is connected to nerve endings, so when something brushes against you (like a mosquito or a crawling insect) you feel it immediately. That rapid detection can trigger a reflex to swat it away, helping prevent bites or the spread of pathogens that insects might carry.

Now take a look inside your nose (well, maybe just imagine it). All those tiny nose hairs? They're not there just to annoy you during allergy season. They serve a filtering function, trapping dust, pollen, mold spores, bacteria, and even viruses before they can make their way deeper into your respiratory system. It's like nature's version of an air purifier—sifting out the bad stuff right at the entrance.

Your eyelashes are also mini gatekeepers, for your eyes. They catch debris, protect against tiny particles in the air, and even help trigger a blinking reflex if something comes too close. That's why you blink if someone pretends to poke your eye, even if they don't touch you!

Your eyebrows do a lot more than give your face character. They help direct sweat, rain, and oil away from your eyes, keeping your vision clear and preventing irritants and potential pathogens from dripping into one of the body's most sensitive orifices.

Inside your ears, you've got tiny hairs that work with earwax to trap unwanted particles like dust, dirt, and small insects. These hairs help form a protective barrier, keeping the eardrum safe and clean.

CILIA

Now here's where it gets super cool, deep inside your bronchial tubes (the airways in your lungs), you've got microscopic hair-like structures called cilia. These aren't hairs in the traditional sense, but they function similarly. They wave rhythmically, almost like seaweed under water, to push mucus (and all the trapped bacteria, viruses, and dust particles) up and out of your lungs.

It's basically a self-cleaning conveyor belt. When you cough or clear your throat, that's the body's way of ejecting all the junk that the cilia have worked hard to gather and move. This keeps your lungs clean and reduces your chances of developing infections like pneumonia or bronchitis.

So, cilia might seem small and insignificant, but it's actually a crucial player in your immune defense system. It detects, filters, traps, and it even helps eject harmful particles from your body.

From the surface of your skin to deep in your lungs, your body is covered, literally and figuratively, by systems designed to *keep you safe* before your immune cells even have to show up to the fight.

MUCOUS MEMBRANES

Your mucous membranes are one of the most underrated, yet incredibly powerful players in your immune system.

We don't usually think much about mucus, unless we're reaching for a tissue during a cold. But that slick, gooey substance (and the tissue it comes from) is doing some serious heavy lifting when it comes to keeping you healthy.

Mucous membranes are the soft, moist linings that cover and protect the inside surfaces of many parts of your body, especially those that are open to the outside world. We're talking nasal passages, mouth and throat, eyelids, lungs, digestive tract, urethra and genitals, etc.

They line these areas with a protective coating of mucus, which is sticky, slippery, and loaded with immune defense tools.

Let's break down exactly what mucous membranes do to protect your health.

Mucus is like flypaper for germs. When viruses, bacteria, or dust particles try to sneak into your body through your nose, mouth, or lungs, mucus traps them. That way, instead of heading deeper into your body, these intruders get *stuck* right at the entryway.

Think of it like a welcome mat, but instead of wiping your feet, pathogens get stopped in their tracks.

Once mucus traps the bad guys, your body works to get rid of them. That could mean:

- Sneezing them out of your nose
- Coughing them out of your throat
- Swallowing mucus so it can be destroyed by your stomach acid
- Or just letting them drip out (not glamorous, but effective!)

It's a self-cleaning system—and it's always on duty.

And mucus isn't just sticky, it's *smart*. It contains immune substances like:

- Antibodies (especially IgA) that neutralize invaders
- Enzymes that break down bacterial cell walls
- Lactoferrin, a protein that starves bacteria of iron

All of this adds up to a *chemical defense line* that supports the physical barrier.

Mucous membranes also keep tissues moist, which is super important. When these linings dry out—say, in cold weather or heated indoor air—they're more prone to cracks or tiny breaks, which can let pathogens slip in. So mucus acts like a moisturizing shield, keeping tissues soft, pliable, and sealed up.

Mucous membranes in your stomach and intestines help block harmful bacteria in food and even trigger immune responses when necessary.

Mucous membranes are like the secret service of your immune system. They block entry points, trap and flush out invaders, neutralize threats with chemical defenses, and maintain the health of your body's most vulnerable openings.

And they do all this *before* your deeper layers of defense ever kick in. That makes them one of the first lines of defense, working 24/7 to keep the rest of your immune system from having to clean up a much bigger mess.

EXCRETION AND EXPULSION

Most people don't immediately think of sweat, vomit, sneezing, or even breath as part of the immune system, but they are all part of a powerful, built-in defense strategy that your body uses constantly to stay healthy. These processes fall under the umbrella of excretion and expulsion, and they're critical for eliminating threats and maintaining balance inside your body.

First, What's the Difference?

Excretion: This is your body's way of removing *internal waste* that builds up as a result of normal metabolic processes. Think: sweat, urine, carbon dioxide.

Expulsion: This refers more to how your body actively pushes out harmful or irritating substances from the digestive or respiratory system — like when you vomit, sneeze, or have diarrhea.

Both are part of your immune system's "cleanup crew."

Let's start with sweat. Most people associate it with just cooling the body, which it does. But it also helps to remove waste products and toxins through the skin… your largest organ!

When you sweat, you're excreting water, but also small amounts of urea, ammonia, salt, and toxins that the body doesn't want hanging around.

The act of sweating flushes out pores, which helps to remove debris and pathogens from the skin's surface.

Sweat also contains antimicrobial peptides like dermcidin, which help kill bacteria and viruses before they can penetrate the skin.

Think of sweating as your body rinsing off its own armor.

Exhaling is another example. When you exhale, you're not just getting rid of carbon dioxide, you're expelling waste that your cells produce during energy metabolism.

Carbon dioxide (CO_2) is acidic and can be harmful if it builds up. Exhaling keeps your internal pH in check — a balance that's essential for immune cells to function properly.

You also exhale *aerosolized particles and moisture,* which may contain tiny pathogens or irritants, especially when your body is trying to clear a respiratory infection.

Ever notice how you breathe harder during a fever? That's your immune system ramping up the removal of heat and waste.

Now let's move onto expulsion.

Vomit isn't pleasant, but it's your body's rapid-response system for dangerous substances.

For example, if you've ingested something toxic, spoiled, or irritating (like harmful bacteria or a virus), your digestive system can trigger vomiting to expel the threat quickly. This reaction is coordinated by your brain, gut, and nervous system — a sign of just how seriously the body takes incoming threats. It's part of the gut's immune defense, where around 70–80% of immune cells reside!

Not fun, but incredibly effective. It's like yanking the fire alarm before the flames spread.

Diarrhea is another case of flushing out pathogens from the intestines. It may be caused by bacteria, viruses, or food that your body recognizes as dangerous. Instead of allowing harmful microbes to stay and replicate, your intestines release extra fluid to literally wash them out. It's uncomfortable, but it minimizes how much time those invaders have to cause damage or infect deeper tissue.

Your body's telling you: "Let's get this out — fast."

Other forms of expulsion are coughing, sneezing, tears, and urination.

Together, all of these excretory and expulsive actions help your immune system.

You see, if your body couldn't sweat, exhale, vomit, or produce diarrhea, toxins and pathogens would build up inside you, weakening your immune response and increasing your risk of disease. These "messy" processes might seem inconvenient, but they're your body's early warning system and sanitation crew, all in one.

TEMPERATURE

Your body has a built-in thermostat which is incredibly smart. Think of your *hypothalamus* (a tiny but powerful part of your brain) as your body's internal *thermostat*. It's constantly monitoring your temperature and adjusting it as needed, like a smart home system that knows when to turn on the heat or A/C depending on what's going on outside.

Now, under normal circumstances, your internal body temperature sits comfortably around 98.6°F (37°C). But when the body senses an invader (like a virus or bacteria) the hypothalamus says, *"Wait a minute, let's make things a little uncomfortable for these guys,"* and raises the temperature.

That's a fever, and it's *not* a malfunction. It's actually one of the most ancient and effective tools your body has for defending itself.

When a fever kicks in, it's not random, it's on purpose. It's slowing down or killing pathogens. Many bacteria and viruses have a hard time surviving in warmer environments. By raising your core temperature, your body is basically saying, *"Let's bake these invaders out."* Viruses replicate more slowly at higher temperatures and bacteria often can't withstand a sustained fever, their growth is inhibited, giving your immune system the upper hand.

Fever boosts your immune warriors. It doesn't just harm the bad guys, it also supercharges your good guys.

White blood cells (WBCs) become more active and move faster when your body is warmer. T cells, which help kill infected cells, respond more aggressively. Antibodies—the proteins your body creates to tag and neutralize invaders—are produced in greater numbers and work more efficiently. Interferons which are proteins that interfere with viral replication, are released more rapidly during a fever.

So, fever is like turning on the emergency lights and hitting the gas pedal, making the immune response faster and stronger.

But the body also knows when to cool itself down. You see, fevers can be powerful, but your body also knows when to put on the brakes. If the temperature gets too high—typically above 104°F (40°C) — it can become dangerous, especially in children or the elderly.

Don't fear though, that's when the hypothalamus steps in again, working with systems like sweating, vasodilation, and increased respiration to lower the temperature and prevent damage to tissues or organs.

In other words, your body knows when to heat up, and when to cool off.

Have you ever wondered why, when you're feeling unwell, there are moments when you feel cold even though your temperature is elevated? In those instances, all you want to do is wrap yourself in layers of blankets. Then, almost suddenly, you find yourself sweating and tossing off every blanket and article of clothing you can.

What's happening in your body during these fluctuations is a natural response to fever and its accompanying temperature regulation. Your body is signaling for your attention. It's working hard to maintain balance. This is a sign of your immune system in action, fighting off the illness.

So, the next time you experience these shifts during a fever, remember: *your body is smart.* Pay attention to its cues, and give it the support it needs to combat whatever you're facing.

Fever and Cancer Prevention: A Fascinating Connection

Here's where it gets even more interesting.

Over the last few decades, researchers have been exploring the link between fever and cancer prevention. While the science is still developing, some recent studies suggest that fevers might play a role in immune surveillance, the body's ability to recognize and eliminate abnormal (potentially cancerous) cells.

Researchers are finding that fever enhances immune surveillance, especially by activating *natural killer (NK) cells* and *cytotoxic T cells*, which are both key players in destroying cancer cells.[1]

A 2020 review in *Frontiers in Oncology* explored how induced hyperthermia (intentionally raising body temperature) is being studied as a *complementary cancer treatment*, particularly for melanoma and prostate cancer.[2]

A 2018 study found that people who experienced frequent, mild fevers in their lifetime had *lower rates of certain cancers*, suggesting that the fever response may help the body "catch and clean up" abnormal cells early.[3]

The use of fever therapy in historical cancer treatments, like the work of Dr. William Coley in the early 1900s, who used bacterial toxins to induce fevers in cancer patients, is gaining renewed interest in immunotherapy circles today.[4]

So, there's growing belief that fever might not just help with fighting infections, but could also prime the immune system to detect and destroy cancer cells before they become dangerous.

Temperature is a tool, not a threat. Think of body temperature like a dial on your immune system. When there's no threat, your thermostat keeps you cozy and stable. But when trouble shows up—a virus, bacteria, or even a potential cancer cell—your body turns up the heat to give itself a tactical advantage.

And best of all? It usually knows when to cool things back down.

So next time you have a fever, rather than seeing it as a problem to squash immediately with drugs, you might think of it as your body doing what it was brilliantly designed to do — fight back.

"Give me a fever and I can cure any illness"
—Hippocrates

ACIDITY

pH (potential hydrogen) is just a fancy way of measuring how acidic or alkaline something is. The scale runs from 0 to 14:

- **0–6** = acidic
- **7** = neutral
- **8–14** = alkaline (or basic)

Now, you might not think of "acidity" as a defense mechanism, but your body does. It uses different pH levels strategically throughout various systems to help guard against pathogens like bacteria, viruses, and parasites.

Let's take a little tour through the body and see how it works.

Your skin is the largest organ of the immune system, and believe it or not, it's slightly acidic. The surface of healthy skin usually sits at a pH of around 4.5 to 5.5.

Why does that matter? Because most harmful microbes, including bacteria and fungi, prefer a more neutral or slightly alkaline environment to thrive. When your skin is acidic, it's like having a protective moat around your castle that makes it really hard for invaders to settle in.

In fact, when you overuse soaps or skincare products that disrupt your skin's natural pH, you can actually make it easier for infections to take hold, that's why the term "acid mantle" is often used to describe this vital, invisible defense layer.

Mucous membranes—in your nose, throat, lungs, gut, and reproductive tracts—are more than just moist tissues. They're part of your first line of defense, and they have their own unique pH zones.

Nasal and respiratory mucus has a slightly acidic pH (around 5.5–6.5) to help trap and neutralize pathogens.

Vaginal mucus is famously acidic (pH ~3.8–4.5) to keep harmful bacteria and yeasts from overgrowing.

Tears and saliva also have slightly acidic to neutral pH, with enzymes like lysozyme that break down bacterial walls.

These pH levels are tailored for maximum pathogen-busting power in each specific area.

Now, let's talk about the real MVP of the body's pH-driven defense system: the stomach.

Your stomach is an acidic inferno, and for good reason. The pH of stomach acid (mostly hydrochloric acid) ranges from **1.5 to 3.5**, which is powerful enough to break down food *and* kill most pathogens that try to sneak in through your mouth.

Ever wonder why we don't get sick every time we eat something questionable? That stomach acid is usually the reason. It kills bacteria like E. coli, Salmonella, and Listeria before they can cause trouble. It helps activate digestive enzymes like pepsin, which break down proteins — part of how your body repurposes what it eats into usable parts. It helps control the gut microbiome, making sure harmful organisms don't outnumber the good ones.

But here's the kicker: when stomach acid is too low (a condition called hypochlorhydria), you're more likely to experience infections, digestive issues, and poor absorption of nutrients. So yes, too much acid can cause problems (hello, heartburn), but too little is also risky from an immune standpoint.

Why does pH matter so much to immunity? Your body uses acidic environments to kill or slow down pathogens. These environments help activate immune cells and enzymes, and disrupted pH balance. Whether from poor diet, stress, medications like antacids, or illness, a disrupted pH can weaken these defenses and make you more vulnerable to infection.

Think of pH as the landscape of your internal terrain. When it's balanced, you're less hospitable to germs and better equipped to fight off illness. When it's off, you're giving the bad guys a better shot (Terrain Theory). pH is an unsung hero!

We often hear about white blood cells, antibodies, and inflammation when we talk about the immune system. But your body's pH balance is like the stage they perform on. If the terrain is set up right, a little acidic here, a little alkaline there, your immune players are set up for success.

So, the next time you think about staying healthy, remember: it's not just what's fighting the germs, it's where the battle takes place.

THE INTERNAL ADAPTIVE IMMUNE SYSTEM

When we talk about the immune system, it's like peeling back layers of an onion. We've already covered the outer layers: your skin, hair, mucus membranes, and things like fever and pH that keep invaders at bay. But let's go all the way in, deep inside your body, to the powerhouse core of your immune defense: the innermost layer made up of white blood cells, antibodies, and a smart communication network called the lymphatic system. This is known as the adaptive immune system.

At the heart of this system are white blood cells, also known as leukocytes. These are like the foot soldiers of your immune army. They're constantly on patrol in your bloodstream, scanning for anything that doesn't belong, like bacteria, viruses, or even mutated cells.

There are different types of white blood cells with different jobs. Some are like the first responders, rushing to the site of an infection and kicking off inflammation to alert the rest of the immune system. Others are more specialized, like detectives and assassins all rolled into one.

Now, let's break it down a bit more. You've got T cells and B cells, which are superstars of the adaptive immune system, the part that learns and remembers.

T cells are like precision fighters. Some of them, called killer T cells, target and destroy infected cells directly. Others, like helper T cells, rally the troops and tell the rest of the immune system what to do. Without them, the response would be chaotic and weak.

B cells have a different role. They're like the intel team. When they recognize an intruder, they start producing antibodies, which are Y-shaped proteins that lock onto specific pathogens like a key fitting a lock. Once antibodies bind to a virus or bacteria, they neutralize it and flag it for destruction.

Now, all of this needs a delivery system, and that's where the *lymphatic system* comes in. Think of it as a hidden highway that runs throughout your body, carrying lymph (a clear fluid full of immune cells) through a series of checkpoints called *lymph nodes*. If you've ever had swollen glands in your neck when you're ill, that's your lymph nodes swelling up while they trap and destroy invaders.

This system helps circulate immune cells where they're needed and filters out dangerous material along the way.

And the coolest part? Once your body successfully fights off a microbe, it doesn't just move on and forget. It *remembers*. Those B cells and T cells form memory cells. If that same germ ever tries to invade again, your immune system recognizes it immediately and launches a faster, stronger attack. That's why you usually only get chickenpox, measles, or mumps once.

So while your outer layers of defense like your skin, hair, mucus and pH do a lot of the heavy lifting to keep germs out, it's the innermost layer, your white blood cells, T cells, B cells, antibodies, and the lymphatic system, that handle the real battles inside your body. This layer is smart, fast, and adaptable. And once it wins a fight naturally, it doesn't forget. Natural Active Immunity makes you *immune for life*.

You see, when we talk about germs or microbes making us sick (germ theory), it almost sounds like they just waltz right into our bodies and start causing chaos. But in reality, it's not even close to that simple. Your body has layer upon layer of tough, smart, and highly coordinated defenses that a microbe has to get through *before* it even has a shot at reaching your inner tissues or bloodstream. And by the time it does (if it even makes it that far), it's usually in rough shape, weakened, broken down, and far easier for your immune system to handle.

This flies in the face of the vaccination paradigm which *injects* the foreign invaders, bypassing all of the layers of defense listed above, and inserts them directly inside your ill-prepared body, along with other immune compromising ingredients and chemicals (to be discussed in later chapters).

So the next time you hear about a "dangerous germ," remember: your body doesn't just sit back and let it run wild. It's a fortress with multiple layers of surveillance, defense, and response. And any microbe that manages to make it deep inside naturally? It's already been through a war, and your immune system is ready to finish the job.

Natural Passive Immunity

Natural passive immunity occurs when immunity (antibodies, WBC's, etc.) is passed from one individual to another naturally, without the recipient's immune system having to produce it.

Natural passive immunity only takes place between mother and child. It is the transfer of ready-made antibodies from a mother to her baby, providing immediate, short-term protection against infections.

During pregnancy, antibodies (mostly IgG) cross the placenta from mother to fetus.

After birth, antibodies (especially IgA) are delivered through breast milk, especially in colostrum, the first milk produced.

"Natural" means it happens without medical intervention. "Passive" means the antibodies are given to the body, not made by it.

Natural passive immunity provides only temporary protection—lasting weeks to months (or years, depending on how long the mother nurses her child) until the baby's own immune system matures.

You've probably heard the phrase "breast is best" at some point, but what's often left out of the conversation is just how intelligent and immune-focused breastfeeding really is. It's not just about nutrition, it's about communication, protection, and *teamwork* between the mother's body and her baby's developing immune system.

From the very first drops of breast milk (called colostrum) a baby is getting far more than calories. Colostrum is thick, golden, and packed with powerful immune components. It's often referred to as "liquid gold" because it's loaded with antibodies, white blood cells, enzymes, and growth factors. These aren't just random ingredients, they're tailored to fight off the very pathogens a newborn might encounter in the outside world.

Most notably, colostrum contains high levels of secretory IgA, a special kind of antibody that lines the baby's digestive tract, helping to block harmful germs from even getting a foothold.

When a baby is born, their immune system is still under construction. They haven't had time to develop their own full set of defenses yet. So breast milk acts like a rented immune system, a beautiful example of what we call natural passive immunity. The mother passes along her own antibodies through her milk, giving the baby targeted, real-time protection against the things *she's already been exposed to.*

So if a mother caught a cold a few months ago and developed antibodies, those exact immune defenses are passed on to her baby through her breast milk. Even if she's simply exposed to microbes, pathogens, or environmental toxins (and doesn't get sick because her internal terrain is strong) she still shares those immunological responses with her child.

That means the baby receives a built-in early-warning system and protective shield, without ever having to suffer through the illness themselves.

So think about it: if mother and baby are together constantly (as they usually are during the nursing months), then mom's immune system becomes the baby's outer fortress wall, standing guard while the infant's own defenses develop, strengthen, and mature.

Now here's where things get *really* amazing—breastfeeding isn't a one-way street. The mother isn't just giving milk, she's actually receiving information from her baby's body too.

When the baby nurses, their saliva is pulled into tiny ducts in the mother's nipple. That's right, the nipple acts like a *two-way communication device.* The baby's saliva contains chemical signals and traces of pathogens or physiological markers. When the mother's body detects something is off, like the baby starting to fight off a cold, it immediately begins adjusting the composition of the milk to meet the child's needs!

That could mean increasing the number of white blood cells in the milk, producing more specific antibodies, or even changing the balance of fats and nutrients to give the baby extra energy to recover. It's like having a real-time, personalized natural pharmacy built into the breastfeeding relationship.

But the benefits don't stop when the baby stops nursing. Breastfeeding actually trains the child's immune system, helping it learn which microbes are threats and how to respond appropriately. Research shows that breastfed babies tend to have fewer respiratory infections, stomach bugs, and even lower risks of allergies and autoimmune issues later in life.

So, in short, breastfeeding is one of the most incredible examples of biological teamwork between two people. It's immune support, custom-tailored nutrition, and communication all rolled into one! And the longer a baby is breastfed, the more opportunities the mother's body has to continue adapting and protecting, like a living, breathing immunological partnership.

Artificial Active Immunity

Artificial active immunity is a type of immunity that develops when a person is exposed to a weakened or inactivated form of a pathogen through medical intervention, such as a vaccine. The body then actively produces its own immune response.

Artificial active immunity is immunity gained through vaccination, hoping that the body is stimulated to create its own defenses against a disease without having to experience the full illness.

"Artificial" means it's introduced by medical means (like a vaccine). "Active" means the body's own immune system responds.

Artificial active immunity may provide temporary protection, which will wane over time, requiring booster shots to maintain effectiveness.

Important Notes:

- Artificial active immunity *does not produce lifelong protection*, unlike natural infections which lead to more durable, long-term immunity. That's why many vaccines are part of a schedule which includes booster doses.

- Vaccines bypass all the outer defenses of the immune system (mentioned above), by injecting foreign substances directly into muscle tissue, as opposed to: Natural infections, in which microbes must pass through all the outer defenses, triggering the body's multi-layered immune defenses. With injections, the immune system is being artificially provoked, with antigens, adjuvants, preservatives, and foreign biological material which cause inflammation and other immune suppressing reactions (discussed in later chapters).
- Artificial Active Immunity is an inherent assault on the body. Put simply, it's immune manipulation. It may also provoke unintended reactions, as we'll discuss and prove in later chapters.

Artificial Passive Immunity

Artificial Passive Immunity is a type of immunity that is acquired by the injection of antibodies into a person's body to help fight off an infection or provide temporary protection against a specific disease.

Artificial Passive Immunity is obtained when *ready-made antibodies*, created outside of the body (usually in a lab or from donor plasma), are given to someone who has either been exposed to a disease, or is at high risk of infection and needs immediate, short-term protection.

Antivenom, Rabies immunoglobulin, Hepatitis B immunoglobulin (HBIG), and Monoclonal antibodies are examples of artificial passive immune methods.

Artificial Passive Immunity is *temporary* because the body is receiving ready-made antibodies from an external source, it's not making them itself. That means the immune system doesn't "learn" or "remember" how to fight the pathogen in the future.

When you're given artificial passive immunity (like an injection of antibodies), it's kind of like borrowing someone else's defense system. Those antibodies will float around in your bloodstream and immediately go to work to neutralize the threat. But, after a few weeks or months, they naturally break down and disappear, just like any protein in the body.

And since your own immune system didn't do the work to make those antibodies, it doesn't remember the infection. So the next time you're exposed to that same pathogen, you're just as vulnerable as before.

The Power of Natural Active Immunity: Lifelong Protection

When it comes to our body's defenses, *not all immunity is created equal*. Out of the four types of immunity—natural and artificial, active and passive— only one stands out for giving us lifelong protection: *Natural Active Immunity*.

As mentioned earlier, this form of immunity develops when your body is exposed to a pathogen naturally (like recovering from chickenpox or the flu).

In response, your immune system: Fights off the invader, Creates antibodies, and most importantly, builds memory cells that "remember" how to respond if the same microbe shows up again—even decades later.

These memory cells last a lifetime, meaning your immune system becomes better and faster at dealing with future exposures.

That's what makes this form of immunity so powerful. And there are no artificial chemicals or ingredients involved!

So while vaccines (Artificial Active Immunity) aim to mimic this process, they don't provide long-term protection—hence the need for boosters. And passive forms of immunity (like antivenoms or maternal antibodies passed to infants) offer only temporary protection and no immune memory.

Chapter Sources

1. Evans, S. S., Repasky, E. A., & Fisher, D. T. (2015). Fever and the thermal regulation of immunity: The immune system feels the heat. *Nature Reviews Immunology, 15*(6), 335–349.
2. van der Zee, J. (2020). Hyperthermia in cancer treatment: Questions remain. *Frontiers in Oncology, 10*, 605711.
3. Zhou, G., & Liao, A. (2018). Fever and cancer incidence: Findings from observational studies. *Medical Hypotheses, 117*, 46–49.
4. Hoption Cann, S. A., van Netten, J. P., & van Netten, C. (2003). Dr William Coley and tumour regression: A place in history or in the future. *Postgraduate Medical Journal, 79*(938), 672–680.

Chapter 4: Truth #2 - Vaccines Don't Build Herd Immunity—They Undermine It

(Temporary protection ≠ lasting public health.)

What Is Herd Immunity?

Let's start simple: herd immunity is the idea that when a large enough portion of a population becomes immune to a disease, the disease has a hard time spreading. That way, even those who aren't immune are less likely to be exposed to the pathogen, and become ill, because the "herd" around them acts as a buffer.

Think of it like this: Imagine you're driving down a busy interstate on a major holiday. It's late, you're exhausted, and all you want is to find a place to rest for the night. But every hotel you pass has a big "No Vacancy" sign. There's simply nowhere for you to stop. So, you're forced to keep moving until eventually, you give up or run out of fuel.

That's how herd immunity works. When the majority of a population becomes immune to a particular microbe, through natural exposure and recovery, it's like hanging a "No Vacancy" sign on most potential hosts. The pathogen can't find enough people to infect, so it has nowhere to settle and multiply. Eventually, it fizzles out, unable to maintain its presence in the population.

The History of the Concept

The idea of herd immunity actually dates back to the early 20th century. The term was first used in medical literature in 1916, but it gained traction in the 1920s and 1930s, particularly in studies of measles and cattle disease.

The earliest observations of herd immunity actually came from veterinary medicine, particularly in livestock, before the concept was widely applied to human populations.

Before scientists fully understood how diseases spread among humans, they were already seeing clear patterns in animal populations, especially cattle and sheep. In the early 1900s, veterinarians and farmers noticed something fascinating: when a large enough portion of a herd recovered from a particular illness, future outbreaks of the same disease seemed to fizzle out quickly, or didn't happen at all.

One of the most cited early examples involved Brucellosis, also known as contagious abortion in cattle. This disease caused pregnant cows to miscarry. In herds where many cows had previously been exposed and recovered, the disease didn't seem to spread again with the same intensity, even when new animals were introduced.

Veterinarians began to realize that recovered animals became naturally immune. When enough animals were immune, outbreaks could no longer spread freely. Then the herd, as a whole, was protected, even if not every single animal had become ill.

This is where the term "herd immunity" began to take shape, literally describing the immunity status of a group or "herd" of animals.

Similar patterns were seen with sheep and swine diseases. For example hoof-and-mouth disease outbreaks would taper off once a certain percentage of hoofed animals had been exposed and developed resistance. Rinderpest, a disease in cattle and buffalo, was also observed to decline when enough animals gained immunity naturally after overcoming the infection.

Farmers, long before formal immunology developed, practiced natural disease control by exposing healthy animals intentionally to other animals who were ill. By allowing herds to cycle through infections and therefore protect the rest in future seasons, the natural decline of the disease from natural active immunity achieved herd immunity.

One of the first scientific observations of herd immunity in humans occurred in 1916 during a measles outbreak in the U.S. Researchers noticed that when a significant portion of children in a community became immune after an outbreak, future outbreaks were milder and shorter—because the disease had fewer people to infect.

In 1933, A.W. Hedrich published a pivotal paper documenting measles patterns in Baltimore. He showed that when around 68% of children were immune, measles outbreaks declined significantly. This was one of the earliest formal introductions of herd immunity thresholds.

The Roots of Herd Immunity: Naturally Strong

It's important to recognize that herd immunity, in its original form, is developed through natural active immunity. That is, when people (or animals) were exposed to a disease, overcame it, and then became permanently immune. This kind of immunity is durable and lifelong, because it involves a full immune response: exposure to the *whole* pathogen, memory cell formation, antibody production, and T-cell activation.

Historically, this is how populations *naturally* developed resistance to diseases. Outbreaks would occur, people would recover, and over time, the community as a whole would become protected because there were fewer and fewer people left for the disease to infect.

With the introduction of vaccines, we saw a shift toward *artificial active immunity*, where a weakened or partial version of a pathogen is introduced to stimulate an immune response. While this sounds ideal in theory, there's a key difference:

- Natural active immunity lasts a lifetime.
- Artificial active immunity is temporary.

This difference matters because *temporary immunity would not sustain herd immunity over time.* If a large portion of the population attempts to rely on vaccines that *wane in effectiveness,* then as time passes, immunity can drop below the threshold needed for herd protection, reopening the door for outbreaks.

Using Critical Thinking to Sort Out Herd Immunity

The vaccine narrative leans heavily on a particular kind of logic: *inductive reasoning.* It goes something like this: during natural outbreaks, when a large number of people get sick and recover, the spread of the disease slows down or stops.

Take measles, for example:

Before widespread vaccination, most kids caught it young, recovered, and came out the other side with lifelong immunity. Eventually, so many had *natural immunity* that outbreaks faded on their own.

So the thinking went, if natural immunity can slow or stop transmission, then we can mimic that effect by artificially creating immunity through vaccines. Just get enough people injected, and voilà, herd immunity.

Sounds tidy. But it's a leap. A big one. And one that doesn't hold up under closer inspection.

That's the trap of inductive reasoning: spotting a pattern, then assuming the pattern explains everything. It's like saying, "I see smoke, so there must be fire," without checking if it's just fog or someone burning toast. Inductive reasoning can suggest possibilities, but it doesn't prove conclusions.

To really test the claim that vaccines create herd immunity, we need to shift from *what seems likely* to *what must logically follow*.

That's deductive reasoning, and it gives us a much clearer picture.

Let's start from the top.

First, artificial immunity, the kind triggered by vaccines, introduces a weakened or partial form of an antigen (virus, bacteria, etc.). It skips most of the body's natural defense mechanisms: the skin, mucous membranes, the digestive tract, etc. The immune system doesn't get the full picture. The result? *A partial immune response*. The body may produce antibodies, but it doesn't go through the entire process that generates durable, long-term memory. Unlike natural infection, vaccine-induced immunity is usually weaker and shorter-lived.

Second, in order to keep that protection going, people have to get booster shots. Repeatedly. But studies show that only about 10 to 15 percent of adults continue to stay "up to date" with boosters after childhood. That means the majority of the population is walking around with waning or expired protection.

Third, real herd immunity, long lasting, population-wide immunity, requires a solid and sustained level of protection across the group. And not just any protection, but the kind that endures. This is exactly what you get when people go through the full immune response that comes from natural infection and recovery. That's how herd immunity actually works. It doesn't rely on constant reactivation. It builds a stable wall.

So here's the conclusion.

If vaccines offer only short-term immunity, and most people don't keep up with their boosters into adulthood, then the vaccinated population gradually loses protection. That leaves *more people vulnerable* over time. And since vaccines have replaced natural exposure in many childhood diseases, those who miss out on lifelong natural immunity are now *more susceptible* as adults. The wall isn't reinforced—it's eroded.

In other words, vaccines don't create herd immunity. They suppress the natural process that builds it. They trade lifelong, natural protection for temporary, artificial coverage. And when that coverage fades, the gaps get bigger, not smaller.

If we follow the logic carefully, we see the flaw. The public health system made an inductive leap, observing that immunity stops disease, and assuming vaccination would do the same. But deductive reasoning reveals a more sobering reality: the kind of immunity matters. And if it's not durable, if it's not complete, then the entire idea of vaccine-induced herd immunity begins to fall apart.

The science isn't settled. The thinking never was.

Disease Decline Before Vaccines

Adding to this conversation is an often-overlooked point, many of the major declines in disease incidence and death occurred *before* vaccines were introduced. Historical public health records show that measles, pertussis, polio, diphtheria, and others saw steep declines due to improvements in sanitation, nutrition, hygiene, and access to clean water. These changes strengthened people's overall health, giving their immune systems a stronger foundation (or "terrain") to naturally fight off infections. As a result, many populations were able to develop Natural Active Immunity, which led to the establishment of Natural Herd Immunity *well before widespread vaccination* campaigns began.

For example, measles mortality dropped by over 98% in the U.S. before the measles vaccine was licensed in 1963.

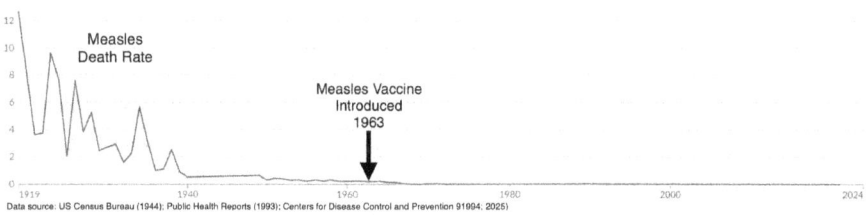

This raises a reasonable question: Was it the vaccine or the environment that really reduced these diseases? And how much of today's disease control should be attributed to immune resilience, societal improvements, and healthy hosts rather than immunization alone? (More on this in the next chapter)

Once again, statistics show that Béchamp's terrain theory stands the test of time, scrutiny, and real life scenarios. Healthier hosts = less disease.

> *The vaccination program is based on the germ theory, a house of cards debunked by Koch's 1st Postulate.*

A Double-Edged Sword?

Based upon the evidence, widespread temporary immunity from vaccines not only does not produce herd immunity, but could actually *suppress* the development of natural herd immunity, leaving the population in a constant cycle of needing boosters and repeat exposures to maintain protection, especially if the vaccine doesn't stop transmission fully or wears off quickly.

In fact, very few people continue with a full vaccine booster schedule throughout their entire lifetime (10-15%).

In contrast, when natural active immunity spreads through a population, it often results in a robust and long-term protection (no boosters needed), helping the disease fade away naturally over time—as seen historically.

The Role of Natural Immunity in Herd Immunity—and How Vaccines Disrupt It

So in summary, herd immunity is supposed to be a population-wide shield. When enough people are immune to a disease, the illness has nowhere to go, and it can't spread. That's the basic idea.

For most of human history, this kind of protection happened naturally. People got exposed, they got sick, they recovered, and they walked away with real, lasting immunity. Not a subscription plan. Just one infection, and the body handled the rest.

The concept of herd immunity didn't come from a lab or a pharmaceutical ad. It came from observing livestock. Farmers noticed that once enough animals caught and beat a disease, outbreaks stopped. The same thing happened in human populations. Before vaccines, illnesses began to fade as large portions of the population gained natural, lifelong immunity. In many cases, both case rates and death rates were already in steep decline *before* vaccines were introduced. Natural exposure was already doing the job.

But modern public health took that principle and tried to repackage it.

Today, herd immunity is sold as something we're supposed to achieve through mass vaccination. But what we're getting isn't real immunity, it's an *imitation*. It's artificial active immunity, and it comes with strings attached.

Unlike natural infection, which activates the entire immune system and creates durable memory, vaccine-induced immunity takes a shortcut. It bypasses the body's normal entry points, and injects lab-made antigens, along with a cocktail of chemicals, metals, genetic material, and adjuvants, directly into the body. This method often produces a weaker immune response. And because it's incomplete, it fades, requiring regular boosters to maintain the illusion of protection.

That leads to a problem. If most people only get this kind of temporary immunity, and if they don't keep showing up for boosters (which most adults don't), then the population isn't actually protected.

We're just going through cycles of fading immunity, followed by urgent calls for more shots. And around we go.

So instead of building toward real, lasting herd immunity, we're interrupting it. Natural immunity is being pushed out of the picture, and in its place, we're left with a fragile, short-lived substitute. The system becomes dependent on artificial stimulation, again and again, just to maintain basic defense. It's not immunity. It's

> **Ironically, rather than building toward true herd immunity, reliance on artificial immunity may suppress the natural development of long-lasting protection, leaving communities dependent on medical intervention indefinitely.**

dependency.

And that dependency just happens to be very, very profitable.

As of 2024, the global vaccine market is worth somewhere between $*70 and $80 billion* (USD)! That's not a typo. Vaccines are one of the most lucrative sectors in the pharmaceutical industry, and they don't just rake in money through the initial childhood series. There's a growing push for adult boosters, travel vaccines, seasonal shots, and "emergency" preparedness injections. The system feeds itself.

Natural immunity, on the other hand, doesn't cost a dime. No appointments. No insurance claims. No cold chain storage or liability waivers. It just works. And once it's in place, it stays in place—providing long-term, lifelong protection, without the need for medical upkeep.

So ask yourself: if real herd immunity can develop naturally, for free, through the body's own design… and vaccine-induced immunity requires endless intervention, constant marketing, and billions in recurring revenue… which one do you think gets promoted?

Natural immunity ends the cycle. Vaccine dependency keeps it spinning.

That's not biology, that's business.

Chapter Sources

1. U.S. Vital Statistics & Historical Data U.S. Department of Health, Education, and Welfare. (1994). *Vital statistics of the United States: Historical trends, 1900–1992.* U.S. Government Printing Office.
2. Thomas McKeown, MD, Epidemiologist McKeown, T. (1976). *The role of medicine: Dream, mirage, or nemesis?* Princeton University Press.
3. CDC Historical Trends Centers for Disease Control and Prevention (CDC). (1999). Achievements in public health, 1900–1999: Control of infectious diseases. *Morbidity and Mortality Weekly Report (MMWR), 48*(29), 621–629.
4. Mortality Trends in Childhood Infectious Diseases Guyer, B., Freedman, M. A., Strobino, D. M., & Sondik, E. J. (2000). Annual summary of vital statistics: Trends in the health of Americans during the 20th century. *Pediatrics, 106*(6), 1307–1317.
5. World Health Organization (WHO) Reports World Health Organization. (n.d.). *Water sanitation and health.*
6. Public Health & Sanitation Literature Szreter, S. (1988). The importance of social intervention in Britain's mortality decline c. 1850–1914: A reinterpretation of the role of public health. *Social History of Medicine, 1*(1), 1–38.

Chapter 5: Truth #3 - Vaccines Didn't Save Us from Disease—We Were Already Winning

(Mortality dropped long before the shots showed up.)

We've all heard the triumphant stories: how vaccines have wiped out deadly diseases and saved humanity from epidemics. It's a tale told with confidence in medical journals, public health campaigns, and classroom textbooks. But what if that story isn't quite so simple… or true?

The Illusion of Eradication — Rethinking Vaccines and Immunity

Despite decades of global vaccination campaigns, the diseases they were meant to conquer are still with us. Some quietly lurking, others reemerging. Boosters are now routine, immunity is temporary, and outbreaks occur even in highly vaccinated populations. And when we step back to look at the broader picture, a more uncomfortable truth begins to emerge: vaccines, as tools of artificial active immunity, may not be eradicating disease at all... but instead prolonging its presence.

Why? Because vaccines often bypass the body's full immune process, offering a partial and short-lived shield. They suppress the natural development of robust, lifelong immunity, the very process that drives true herd immunity. While nature builds durable defenses through exposure and recovery, artificial intervention provides weaker protection that fades, requiring repeated doses to maintain any potential effect.

What's even more striking, is that historical data reveals a consistent pattern: *the steepest declines in disease mortality occurred before the introduction of vaccines,* thanks to naturally induced herd immunity, improved living conditions, nutrition, sanitation, and access to clean water. In contrast, once vaccines entered the scene, they began prolonging, not eliminating, disease.

This chapter explores what few are willing to ask: Have vaccines, in their quest to dominate infectious disease, actually stalled the natural decline of illness? And if so, what does that mean for the future of public health?

If we are to understand the true role vaccines have played in shaping modern disease patterns, we must remember the fundamental distinction: Natural Active Immunity versus Artificial Active Immunity. Let's briefly review:

Natural active immunity is the gold standard of immune protection. It occurs when the body encounters a pathogen, fights it off using the full depth of its multilayered defense system, and then stores the memory of that encounter in specialized immune cells (chapter 3).

This process not only neutralizes the threat, but builds a lifelong immunity. When enough individuals in a population gain this kind of robust protection, true *herd immunity* develops naturally (chapter 4). It's resilient. It's enduring. And historically, it has contributed to the natural decline and even disappearance of many infectious diseases.

Now consider the vaccine model: artificial active immunity. This approach attempts to mimic natural infection by introducing weakened, inactivated, or partial elements of a pathogen, bypassing several critical immune defenses. The immune system responds, but often only partially. And because of this impermanence, we now live in an era which advocates endless boosters and routine re-vaccination.

Here lies the paradox: the more we rely on artificial immunity, the more we interfere with the population's ability to establish long-term, natural protection. The window of temporary immunity offered by vaccines often closes just as individuals reach adulthood, leaving them vulnerable, sometimes more so than those who never received a vaccine in the first place. Children receive dozens of doses during their most formative years, building a foundation of weak, short-term defenses that gradually fade, making the population more susceptible over time unless reinoculated continually.

Meanwhile, pathogens continue to circulate. Not because they're necessarily more virulent, but because the population's immunity is being artificially sustained and allowed to wane, preventing true herd immunity from being genuinely earned and reinforced.

In the coming sections, we'll examine the history and data behind this unsettling dynamic. We'll explore how disease mortality sharply declined before vaccines were introduced. We'll investigate vaccine failure and waning immunity, and how outbreaks occur among vaccinated populations. And most critically, we'll ask: *Have we been solving the wrong problem in the wrong way for far too long?*

Because if we are to move forward with a public health strategy that truly values resilience, we must begin to question whether our current dependence on artificial immunity has hindered, rather than helped, the natural course of disease eradication.

Let's walk through the evidence and consequences of this paradox: that vaccines, intended to eradicate disease, may in fact prolong its presence.

The Disruption of Natural Immune Cycles

Before widespread vaccination programs, communities were exposed to various childhood diseases like measles, mumps, rubella, and chickenpox. These infections, while uncomfortable and rarely serious, resulted in *lifelong immunity* once recovered. This meant that individuals were permanently protected and also contributed to herd immunity by becoming immune buffers, essentially blocking the microbe's path to new, unprotected hosts.

Vaccination programs *interrupted this cycle*. By replacing natural exposure with artificial, partial exposure, they changed how immunity developed across generations. Children, who would once gain permanent immunity through natural recovery, are now given weak, temporary protection that fades. If boosters are not maintained (and most are not) these individuals become susceptible again later in life, sometimes at ages when the same diseases pose *greater risks.* This is particularly true for diseases like measles and chickenpox, which are more severe in adults than in children.

The Artificial Herd Immunity Illusion

Public health authorities often cite herd immunity thresholds (like 95% vaccine coverage) as necessary to prevent outbreaks. But here's the catch: this model only works if the vaccine confers strong and lasting immunity. They do not! The immunity provided by vaccines wanes over time, sometimes significantly within just a few years. This means that even if 95% of the population were vaccinated as children, the percentage of adults who remain protected may be far below herd immunity levels.

> Outbreaks still occur— *many times within highly vaccinated populations*—which raises serious questions about the durability and reliability of vaccine-induced immunity.

This reliance on temporary immunity makes the idea of achieving true herd immunity through vaccines not only fragile but unsustainable. It creates a moving target: immunity coverage today does not guarantee protection tomorrow. Outbreaks still occur, *many times within highly vaccinated populations,*[1,2,3,4] which raises serious questions about the durability and reliability of vaccine-induced immunity.

When Vaccines Delay Disease Rather Than Prevent It

There's growing recognition that vaccination programs may simply be postponing outbreaks rather than preventing them. Take pertussis (whooping cough) as a case in point. Once a routine childhood illness with lifelong immunity post-recovery, today we see cycles of resurgence, even in countries with high vaccination rates. Why? Because the vaccine's protection fades, and natural exposure no longer boosts adult immunity. The result: adults and even infants, who are most at risk, are increasingly vulnerable.

This pattern isn't limited to pertussis. Measles, mumps, and even varicella (chickenpox) have all demonstrated similar post-vaccine shifts in epidemiology, including increased cases among vaccinated individuals, unexpected adult outbreaks, and in some cases, a redefinition of the disease's natural lifecycle.

Vaccines and the Myth of Eradication

While vaccines are often credited with the eradication of diseases, a closer look reveals that disease mortality was already declining, often dramatically, before vaccines were introduced. Graphs of measles and diphtheria mortality in the U.S. and Europe show steep downward trends well before the arrival of their respective vaccines.

These historical patterns suggest that, rather than eradicating disease, vaccines may have simply stepped in at the tail end of a natural decline already in progress.

A Closer Look at the Numbers: Declines That Came Before the Needle

Before the first vaccines were introduced for many of the diseases we associate with immunization campaigns—measles, diphtheria, pertussis (whooping cough), and even polio—something remarkable had already begun to happen: *the cases and death rates of these diseases were plummeting.*

And this wasn't a mild dip, it was a steep, sustained decline, observable in public health records across industrialized nations.

Decades before the widespread implementation of vaccinations, improved sanitation, nutrition, housing, access to clean water, and public health education had already begun transforming the *terrain* of human health which resulted in the natural decline of the disease.

The body, when supported by a strong immune system and healthy environment, was becoming increasingly capable of fighting off infections naturally. In other words, the internal conditions—what many now refer to as the "terrain"—were changing.

This data poses a critical question: If the diseases were already on the decline, how much credit can vaccines genuinely claim?

And even more important: If we had already begun to achieve natural herd immunity and sustainable public health improvements, did we ever need to rely so heavily on artificial interventions in the first place?

Evidence from History: Disease by Disease

To answer these questions, let's examine historical health records and mortality charts for several key illnesses. What you'll see is clear and compelling:

- Measles mortality dropped dramatically in the decades before the measles vaccine was introduced in the 1960s.
- Diphtheria deaths had already plummeted by the time its vaccine arrived.
- Pertussis cases saw a significant reduction due to improved living conditions, long before routine childhood immunization.
- Even polio, once feared for its potential to cause paralysis, was on a steady decline, with better hygiene and nutrition playing significant roles.

These patterns are not anomalies. They're consistent across multiple diseases, countries, and timeframes.

In the following pages, we will walk through each disease, supported by historical data, mortality records, and vaccination timelines. These aren't conspiracy theories or fringe interpretations, they're observations grounded in official public health records, often from the very institutions that promote vaccination today.

The goal is to reframe the narrative with complete context. Because when we understand the full picture, including the power of natural immunity and environmental health, we're better equipped to make truly informed decisions about how best to protect ourselves and future generations.

Let's begin with measles, the disease that has often been held up as the poster child for vaccination success.

Measles: A Decline in Progress Long Before the Vaccine

Measles has often been cited as a leading example of vaccine success. Public health campaigns worldwide have heralded the measles vaccine, introduced in 1963, as the turning point in defeating this childhood illness.

But a closer look at the historical data tells a different story.

By the time the measles vaccine was rolled out, measles mortality in the United States had already declined by over 95% from its peak in the early 20th century. This downward trend began in the late 1800s and continued steadily through the 1950s. The introduction of better nutrition, especially increased access to vitamin A, and clean drinking water, combined with improved living conditions, dramatically strengthened children's ability to recover from measles infections.

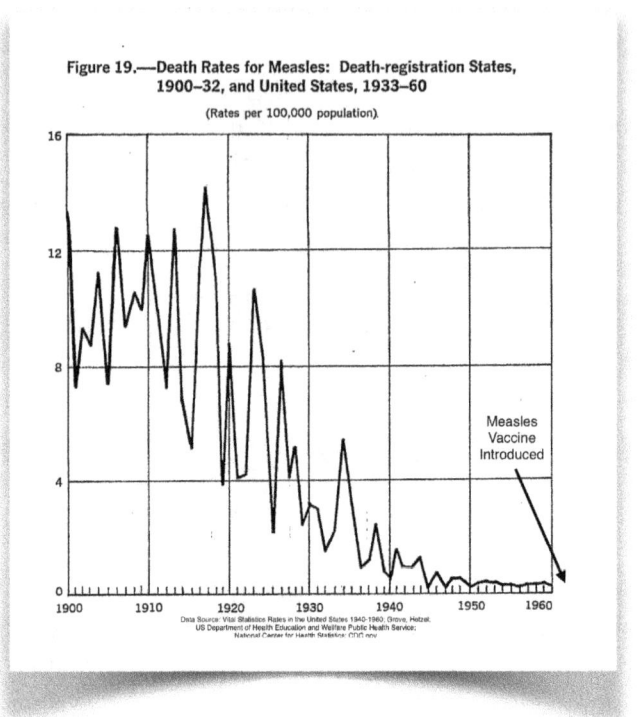

Figure 19.—Death Rates for Measles: Death-registration States, 1900–32, and United States, 1933–60

By the mid-20th century (before the vaccine) most children who contracted measles experienced only mild symptoms and recovered quickly, gaining robust lifelong natural immunity in the process.

Pertussis (Whooping Cough): The Terrain Shifts Before the Shot

Similar patterns were observed with *pertussis*, or whooping cough. In the early 1900s, this disease was a major concern, especially for infants. However, between 1900 and the introduction of the pertussis vaccine in the 1940s, mortality from whooping cough had already dropped by over *75%*.

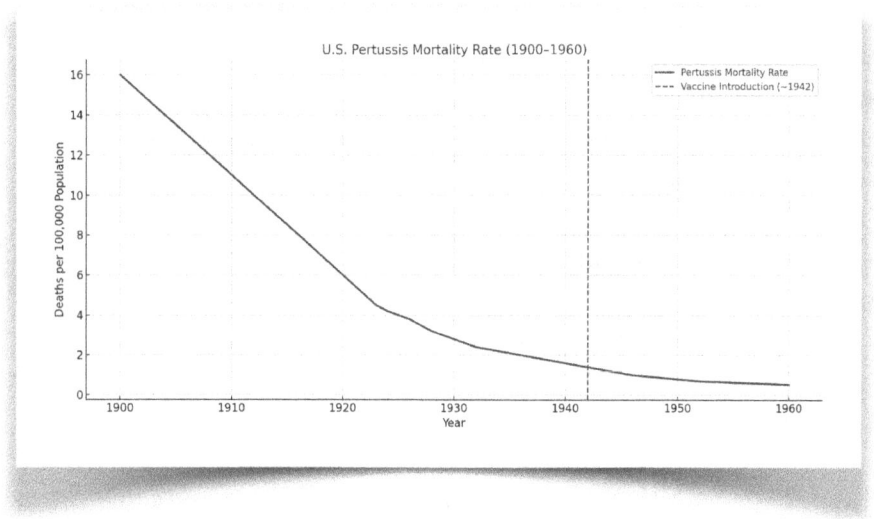

What changed? Once again, it wasn't medicine—it was the *terrain*. Clean water. Sanitation. Increased awareness of the importance of nutrition and hygiene. These societal shifts had a powerful, measurable impact on public health.

What's more, early versions of the pertussis vaccine were plagued with *adverse effects and inconsistent efficacy,* leading to frequent reformulations and booster recommendations. Yet the disease never disappeared, despite decades of mass vaccination.

Diphtheria: Another Example of Premature Credit

Diphtheria was once one of the most feared childhood diseases, known for its thick, choking throat membrane and the terrifying possibility of suffocation. In the late 1800s, it was a leading cause of death in children, especially in crowded cities. It's no wonder people were desperate for a solution.

But here's the part of the story that rarely gets told.

The death rate from diphtheria had already been dropping like a rock long before the vaccine entered the picture. In fact, the majority of the decline had nothing to do with vaccination at all.

In the late 19th century, diphtheria was killing more than 200 people per 100,000 in some U.S. cities. But by 1900, thanks to sweeping improvements in living conditions, nutrition, sanitation, and basic healthcare, the tide was already turning. The bodies getting sick were becoming stronger. The terrain was improving.

By the time the diphtheria toxoid vaccine was introduced in 1923, mortality rates had already fallen by around 60 to 70 percent from their peak. And by 1945, more than 85 percent of the total mortality decline had already occurred.

Let that sink in. The vast majority of lives saved from diphtheria were saved *before* widespread vaccination efforts began.

So what changed?

The answer isn't locked in a syringe. It's in the pipes, the kitchens, and the neighborhoods. Indoor plumbing replaced outhouses. Milk was pasteurized. Nutrition improved as people gained access to fresher, more balanced food. Ventilation in homes and schools got better. Public health campaigns taught basic hygiene, things like handwashing and not spitting in the street. All which led to a natural herd immunity.

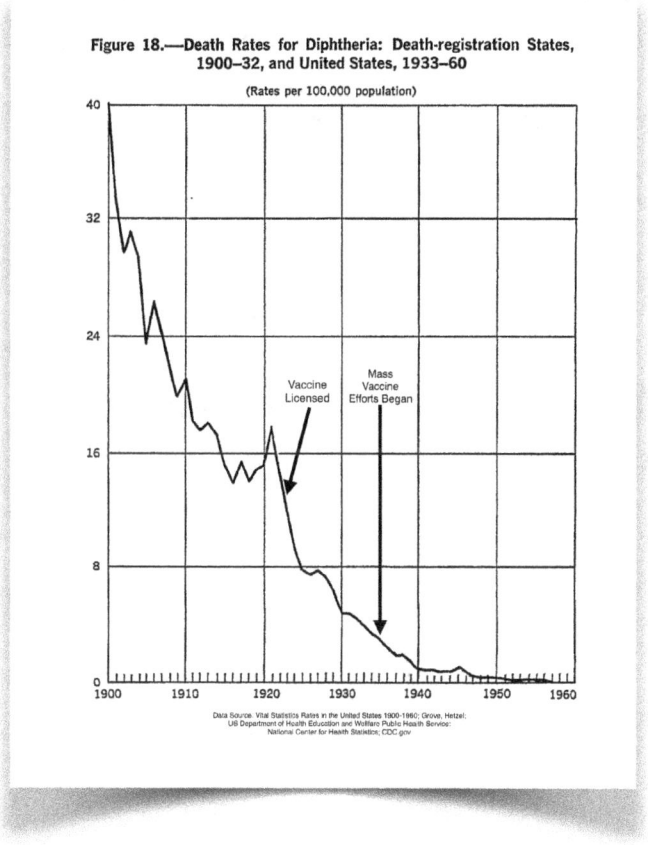

Figure 18.—Death Rates for Diphtheria: Death-registration States, 1900–32, and United States, 1933–60

These are the unsung heroes of the diphtheria story. They don't make headlines. They don't get patented. But they worked.

Historical records and public health data all tell the same story: vaccines were not the primary reason diphtheria mortality dropped. They were introduced after the fact, riding the coattails of improvements that were already doing the heavy lifting.

And that brings us to the larger truth. The body's ability to overcome infection isn't just about killing germs. It's about strengthening the terrain. A well-nourished, well-supported immune system, combined with clean living conditions and real education, can do more to stop disease than a shot ever could.

Once again, the data reinforces what we've explored in depth in Chapter 2: the germ may be the opportunist, but the terrain is the cause. When the terrain improves, disease retreats. And no industry profits from that.

Polio: The Most Feared, But Also Most Misunderstood

While the fear campaigns evoke powerful emotional memories of paralysis and pictures of iron lungs, most polio infections, over 90%, are asymptomatic or mild.

Polio primarily spreads through the fecal-oral route and can lead to flu-like symptoms, and only in some rare cases, paralysis. It most often affected young children, especially in areas with *poor sanitation.*

Polio: Understanding the *Real* Risk

Polio has long been portrayed as one of the most terrifying diseases of the 20th century. While it's true that polio *can* cause paralysis and even death in rare cases, the reality (as stated by the Centers for Disease Control and Prevention) is that for most people, polio is a mild illness.

Let's break this down:

Most polio infections are mild or even asymptomatic. According to the CDC:

- 72% of people infected with poliovirus experience no symptoms at all.
- About 24% develop mild, flu-like symptoms such as:
    - Fever
    - Fatigue
    - Nausea
    - Sore throat
    - Headache

These symptoms *typically go away on their own,* often without the person even realizing they had polio.

Paralysis: The Exception, Not the Rule

- Fewer than 1% of polio infections ever led to paralysis.
- Of those 1% paralytic cases, only a *small fraction* of those resulted in death.

Polio-Related Deaths Are Extremely Rare

- The CDC estimates that among the 1% of people with *paralytic polio:*

    - 2% to 5% of those children may die (that's only 0.02% - 0.05% of overall polio cases).
    - 15% to 30% of those adults, particularly those with breathing muscle involvement, may die (that's only 0.15% - 0.3% of overall polio cases).

Here's what this looks like visually, using **100,000 hypothetical polio cases**:

Outcome	Number of Cases (Estimates)
Asymptomatic	72,000
Mild flu-like symptoms	24,000
Paralysis	<1,000
Death (from paralysis)	~20–50

In other words, over 99% of people infected with poliovirus will recover completely, often without even knowing they were infected!

Why does this matter? Because understanding these numbers is key to a balanced discussion about things like public health policy, vaccine necessity, risk vs. benefit analysis, informed consent, etc.

Polio was serious for only a small percentage of people it affected severely, but for the overwhelming majority, it was a mild, self-limiting illness, not the universal threat it's often portrayed to be.

Polio Mortality and Case Trends Before the Vaccine
- Early 1900s: Sporadic outbreaks began increasing, peaking in the 1940s and early 1950s.
- By 1952, the U.S. reported its largest polio epidemic with over 57,000 cases, but deaths were already declining compared to prior decades.
- The Salk polio vaccine was introduced in 1955.
- Sabin's oral polio vaccine (OPV) followed in 1961.
- By the late 1960s, polio was almost eradicated in the U.S.

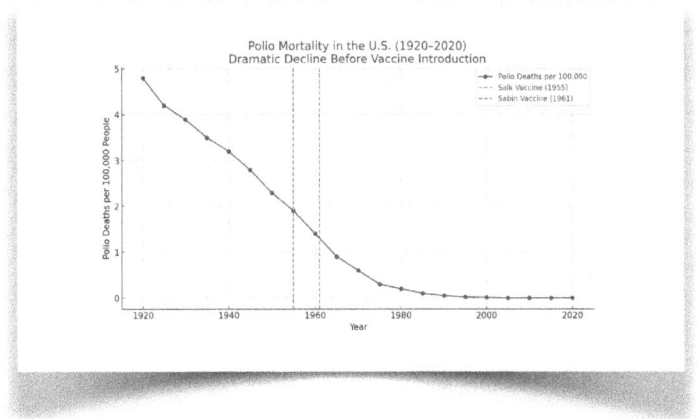

However, this narrative isn't the full picture.

We cannot miss the most important detail: Polio's mortality was already declining before the vaccine introduction.

Changes in Polio Case Definition

One of the most critical and often overlooked issues is that how polio was diagnosed changed significantly after the vaccine was introduced:

- Pre-1955: Any paralytic illness lasting 24 hours could be labeled as polio.
- Post-1955: Paralysis had to last 60+ days, and lab confirmation of the virus was required.

This resulted in an immediate and sharp statistical drop in reported polio cases.

Some researchers argue this reclassification made the vaccine appear more effective than it was.

What Contributed to Polio's Decline (Besides Vaccines)?
- Improved hygiene and sanitation dramatically reduced viral spread.
- Water treatment and sewage systems helped eliminate fecal-oral transmission.
- Better nutrition helped immune resilience in children.
- Natural herd immunity which led to the polio rate drop before widespread vaccine access.

Wild Polio vs. Vaccine-Derived Polio: Understanding the Shift

While wild poliovirus was once a feared and devastating disease, it's important to recognize that the last case of wild polio virus in the United States was reported in 1979. This marked a major milestone in disease control and as the trends and statistics show, natural active immunity and it's resulting natural herd immunity can be cited as the source of victory for polio.

However, the story doesn't end there.

Polio Today: Not Wild, but Vaccine-Derived

According to the Centers for Disease Control and Prevention (CDC) and the World Health Organization (WHO), the only cases of polio now occurring in the Western Hemisphere, including the United States, are no longer from the original wild virus. Instead, they are *caused by the vaccine itself!*

These are known as:

Vaccine-Derived Poliovirus (VDPV)

- The Oral Polio Vaccine (OPV) contains a weakened, live virus.
- This weakened virus can mutate, regain strength, and begin to circulate.
- This mutated strain can then cause outbreaks of vaccine-derived polio.

In other words, the vaccine that was supposed to stop polio has become, in some rare but significant cases, the only source of new polio infections.

Key Points to Understand

Type of Polio	Caused by	Status in the U.S.
Wild Polio Virus	Naturally occurring virus	**Eradicated since 1979**
Vaccine-Derived Polio Virus (VDPV)	Mutation from oral polio vaccine	**Current source of cases**

This phenomenon highlights a *complex irony*: the vaccine was designed to eradicate the wild virus, but today the only cases of polio in the Western Hemisphere are from the vaccine itself, not from natural transmission.

It also underscores the risk of using live-virus vaccines in global programs, particularly in areas with poor sanitation and living conditions.

Post-Vaccine Polio-Like Paralysis

Despite vaccine introduction:

- Vaccine-derived polio (VDPV) became a recognized issue, especially from oral vaccines.

- Acute Flaccid Paralysis (AFP) and other polio-like syndromes (like Guillain-Barré Syndrome) have seen increases post-vaccine, especially in developing countries.

Conclusion: Vaccines Were a Factor, Not the Solution

By the time polio vaccines became widespread in the late 1950s and early 1960s, outbreaks had already started declining in many regions. The major decline in severity, mortality, and transmission of polio occurred:

- *Before* mass vaccination,
- Alongside changes in case definitions, and
- Through public health improvements.

This pattern mirrors that of diphtheria and supports the conclusion that *Natural Active Immunity*, paired with better public infrastructure, was a major force behind polio's decline, long before vaccines.

A Pattern Emerges

Across all these examples, the pattern is striking: *The greatest declines in cases and deaths from infectious diseases occurred before vaccines were introduced.*

Moreover, the introduction of vaccines shifted the landscape of immunity from natural active immunity—which results in lifelong protection and contributes to true herd immunity—to artificial active immunity, which is temporary, incomplete, and requires constant boosting.

And as we will explore in the next section, this shift has not been without unintended consequences.

The Bigger Picture: Public Health or Profitable Dependency?

Artificial immunity requires maintenance—repeat doses, regular boosters, new formulations. This ongoing dependency has created a market worth billions of dollars annually. And while profit alone does not invalidate public health tools, it does raise ethical questions: Are we prioritizing interventions that generate revenue over those that build long-term, resilient health?

Is it truly in the public's best interest to be dependent on scheduled medical intervention from cradle to grave for immunity? Or should we be focusing on strengthening natural immunity through healthier environments, better nutrition, and strategic support of the body's own defenses?

In the final part of this chapter, we'll explore what a health system rooted in natural resilience could look like—and how acknowledging the limits of artificial immunity could shift our approach from one of dependency to one of empowerment and biological integrity.

Let's continue by examining what's at stake when an entire system of immunity relies on artificial support, and what we stand to gain by revisiting the natural immune model that guided humanity for millennia.

A Dependency Model: Immunity on a Timer

Artificial active immunity—by design—requires regular maintenance. The temporary nature of many vaccines means immunity is not a one-and-done outcome, but a time-sensitive effect. Booster shots are required to "remind" the immune system of the pathogen, essentially functioning like periodic system updates.

This dependency model introduces a cascade of consequences:

- **Missed boosters** can lead to vulnerability.
- **Waning immunity** can result in adult outbreaks of childhood diseases.
- **New variants** may not be effectively targeted by existing vaccines, rendering older doses obsolete.

Instead of fostering *biological strength*, we've created a system that depends on consistent external intervention—one that's only as strong as its last injection. This paradigm isn't inherently evil, but it's fragile, resource-intensive, and ignores the body's innate capacity to build long-term defenses when supported properly.

Nature's Blueprint: Self-Sustaining Immunity

Contrast this with natural active immunity, where exposure to a wild pathogen stimulates a full, multilayered immune response—activating the skin and mucosal barriers, triggering inflammation, recruiting white blood cells, and prompting the adaptive immune system to create memory cells. These memory cells provide lifelong immunity.

The brilliance of this system is not only its effectiveness, but its sustainability. Once established, natural immunity:

- Requires no further intervention
- Strengthens the immune system's memory and adaptability
- Contributes to herd immunity without repeat dosing
- Promotes a resilient population that's better prepared for new microbial threats

This is the immunity model that shaped human evolution. It is also the model that allowed disease to burn out in populations historically, leading to long periods of low transmission or eradication—even before vaccines were introduced.

Herd Immunity: Strengthened or Suppressed?

As we've seen, the original concept of herd immunity was rooted in natural infection and recovery (chapter 4). It described the threshold at which enough individuals had encountered and overcome a disease to prevent further spread. It was observational, and not artificially induced.

This is the paradox at the heart of modern immunology: we have confused short-term control with long-term success. In doing so, we may have sacrificed resilience for convenience, and the true cost of that trade is only beginning to reveal itself.

The Hidden Cost of Boosters: Repetition and Ingredients Matter

While boosters are promoted as a simple "tune-up" for the immune system, the frequency and composition of these injections raise valid concerns—especially when considered over a lifetime.

Artificial active immunity, by its very nature, doesn't last. It often fails to produce the deep, lifelong memory that natural infection does. That's why public health protocols recommend multiple doses throughout childhood, adolescence, and even adulthood—culminating in dozens of injections just to maintain a baseline level of protection.

But the issue isn't just the quantity. It's also the quality of what's being injected.

Many booster shots—and the vaccines they're derived from—contain additional ingredients called adjuvants, preservatives, stabilizers, and solvents. These are included not to provoke a direct immune response against a pathogen, but to amplify, preserve, or transport the vaccine's active components. Over time, repeated exposure to these compounds, especially during crucial immune development stages in infants and children, may have cumulative effects that warrant far more scrutiny.

Some common vaccine ingredients that raise concern include:

- Aluminum salts – used as adjuvants to boost immune response, but associated with neurotoxicity and immune dysregulation in high doses or with accumulation.
- Formaldehyde – a known carcinogen used to inactivate viruses and detoxify bacterial toxins.
- Phenoxyethanol – used as a preservative, linked to skin irritation and potential developmental toxicity in animal studies.
- Polysorbate 80 – an emulsifier that may increase blood-brain barrier permeability.
- Thimerosal (ethylmercury) – used as a preservative in multi-dose vials, phased out in some vaccines, but still present in other formulations and in global use.

Regulatory agencies claim these ingredients are used in trace amounts considered safe for human exposure. However, these safety assessments are often conducted on individual ingredients in isolation, not in combined formulations administered repeatedly over years—or even decades.

This is where the problem lies.

Repeated injections, especially starting at birth and continuing throughout life, can lead to bioaccumulation—a slow, persistent buildup of substances in the body. And when substances with potential immune-suppressing, neurotoxic, or inflammatory effects accumulate, it raises the question: *Are we unintentionally weakening the very system we aim to protect?*

A System Strained, Not Strengthened

The irony of it all is that while artificial immunity claims to protect the immune system, it may, over time, actually dull its sharpest edges. By bypassing the skin, mucosa, and digestive barriers—the body's first lines of defense—vaccines are injected directly into tissue and bloodstream, activating an immune response in a disjointed and incomplete way.

Combine that with immune-disruptive ingredients and a lifetime regimen of boosters, and you get an immune system trained to respond artificially, inconsistently, and temporarily.

Natural active immunity, by contrast, teaches the body to fight thoroughly, holistically, and with long-term retention. It doesn't depend on chemical shortcuts—it builds biological intelligence.

So, the next time we're told that "you're due for another booster," we might do well to ask: *What are we boosting—and at what cost?*

The Booster Burden: Repeating Doses, Accumulating Risks

As we've established, artificial active immunity through vaccines does not mirror the lifelong protection of natural active immunity. Unlike immunity acquired through direct exposure and recovery, vaccine-induced immunity often wanes over time —

sometimes in just a few months or years. This leads to the now-familiar concept of booster shots.

Why Boosters?

A booster shot is not a "bonus" dose — it is a necessary reactivation of a fading, weak immune response. This is because the immunity generated by vaccines, particularly in childhood, often does not persist into adulthood without ongoing reinforcement.

In practical terms, this means the very people vaccinated as children may enter adulthood without meaningful protection, unless they continue to receive boosters. However, real-world data shows that only a small fraction of the population maintains up-to-date booster schedules into adulthood. Studies estimate that fewer than 10–15% of adults stay current with recommended boosters. The majority, therefore, carry no reliable immunity despite prior vaccination.

The Repeated Dose Dilemma

Beyond the issue of fading immunity lies another concern: accumulative exposure. With every booster, the body is not only re-exposed to viral or bacterial components — it also receives repeated doses of adjuvants, preservatives, and other additives. While each individual dose may fall within "safe" regulatory thresholds, the cumulative effect of dozens of injections over a lifetime — particularly in developing immune systems — raises significant questions.

While defenders of vaccine safety argue that these ingredients are present in minuscule amounts, critics point out that no other medical intervention is delivered in such frequency, directly into tissue, often bypassing the body's first lines of defense like the skin, mucosa, and gut, and are without risk.

Furthermore, vaccine schedules have dramatically expanded over recent decades. A child in the 1980s received roughly 10 vaccine doses by age 5. Today, many children receive over 70 doses by the time they're 18. This increase is not only in number, but in earlier and more frequent exposures, beginning at birth with the hepatitis B vaccine — a disease rarely encountered by infants outside specific risk categories.

The Paradox: Weak Immunity, Repeated Exposure

This brings us to an important paradox: *If immunity gained through vaccines is so effective, why is it so fragile?*

Natural immunity is robust and durable, often lifelong. But vaccine-induced immunity fades, requiring constant boosting — and with each booster, the risk of immune system fatigue or dysregulation potentially increases.

In some cases, such repeated stimulation may disrupt the immune system's balance, leading to unintended effects such as:

- Autoimmune disorders
- Chronic inflammation
- Reduced ability to respond to natural infections

- Immune suppression, especially in individuals with underlying vulnerabilities

What's more, by substituting artificial exposure for natural infection, the population is no longer building durable herd immunity through natural recovery — a process that once contributed to the eventual natural decline of many diseases.

Instead, the reliance on short-term immunity may have extended the lifespan of diseases that would otherwise have faded more rapidly in a population with robust terrain and strong natural immune memory.

Chapter Sources

1. Gahr, P., DeVries, A. S., Wallace, G., Miller, C., Kenyon, C., Sweet, K., ... & Lynfield, R. (2014). *An outbreak of measles in an undervaccinated community.* Pediatrics, 134(1), e220–e228.
2. Clemmons, N. S., Wallace, G. S., Patel, M., & Gastañaduy, P. A. (2017). *Incidence of measles in the United States, 2001–2015.* JAMA, 318(13), 1279–1281.
3. Gellin, B. G., Maibach, E. W., & Marcuse, E. K. (2000). *Do parents understand immunizations? A national telephone survey.* Pediatrics, 106(5), 1097–1102.
4. World Health Organization (WHO). (2017). Measles outbreaks still a threat despite progress.
5. Centers for Disease Control and Prevention. (n.d.). *Polio – What is polio?* U.S. Department of Health & Human Services.
6. World Health Organization. (n.d.). *Poliomyelitis.*
7. Mayo Clinic. (n.d.). *Polio – Symptoms and causes.*
8. Centers for Disease Control and Prevention. (n.d.). *CDC vaccine timeline and archives.*
9. U.S. Congress, House of Representatives, Committee on Interstate and Foreign Commerce. (1962). *Hearings before the Subcommittee on Health: Poliomyelitis vaccine* (Testimony by Dr. Bernard Greenberg). U.S. Government Printing Office.
10. Blaylock, R. L. (n.d.). The truth behind the vaccine cover-up. Blaylock Wellness Report.
11. Neustaedter, R. (2002). The vaccine guide: Making an informed choice. North Atlantic Books.
12. National Vaccine Information Center. (n.d.). *Disease surveillance and diagnostic shifts.*

13. Centers for Disease Control and Prevention. (2021). *Adult vaccination coverage, National Health Interview Survey, 2021*. U.S. Department of Health & Human Services.
14. Lu, P.-J., O'Halloran, A., Williams, W. W., Lindley, M. C., Farrall, S., & Bridges, C. B. (2017). Adult vaccination coverage—United States, 2015. *American Journal of Preventive Medicine, 53*(6), 872–884.
15. National Foundation for Infectious Diseases. (n.d.). *Adult immunization resources*.
16. U.S. Bureau of the Census. (1975). Historical statistics of the United States: Colonial times to 1970. U.S. Government Printing Office.
17. Centers for Disease Control and Prevention. (1999). Achievements in public health, 1900–1999: Control of infectious diseases. *Morbidity and Mortality Weekly Report, 48*(29), 621–629.
18. McKeown, T. (1976). The role of medicine: Dream, mirage or nemesis? Princeton University Press.
19. Centers for Disease Control and Prevention. (2021). Epidemiology and prevention of vaccine-preventable diseases (The Pink Book). U.S. Department of Health & Human Services.
20. United Kingdom Ministry of Health. (1900–1950). Annual reports on public health and vital statistics.
21. U.S. Bureau of the Census. (1975). Historical statistics of the United States: Colonial times to 1970 (Series B 135–166). U.S. Government Printing Office.
22. National Office of Vital Statistics. (Various years). *Vital statistics of the United States*.
23. Armstrong, G. L., Conn, L. A., & Pinner, R. W. (1999). Trends in infectious disease mortality in the United States during the 20th

century. *Journal of the American Medical Association, 281*(1), 61–66.
24. U.S. Department of Health, Education, and Welfare. (1937–1965). *Vital statistics of the United States* (Annual reports). National Center for Health Statistics.
25. Centers for Disease Control and Prevention. (n.d.). CDC WONDER: Wide-ranging online data for epidemiologic research.
26. Centers for Disease Control and Prevention. (n.d.). *National Notifiable Diseases Surveillance System (NNDSS)*.
27. Hinman, A. R., & Orenstein, W. A. (2004). The immunization system in the United States: The role of school immunization laws. *Vaccine, 22*(15–16), 1390–1396.
28. Neustaedter, R. (2002). The vaccine guide: Making an informed choice. North Atlantic Books.
29. National Center for Health Statistics. (2004). *Health, United States, 2004* (Table 27). U.S. Department of Health & Human Services.

Chapter 6: Truth #4 - The "Safe and Effective" Mantra Is a Marketing Line—Not Science

(Look closer. The studies don't say what you think they do.)

Vaccines have been touted as one of the most significant advancements in public health, credited with reducing, and in some cases eliminating, many deadly infectious diseases. Nonetheless, as discussed in the previous chapter, this may not hold true.

Like any medical intervention, vaccines have been the subject of, not only effectiveness, but also safety concerns, from isolated adverse events to broader questions about ingredients, long-term effects, and cumulative exposure over time.

Examining Vaccine Safety — Understanding the Concerns

In this chapter, we'll take a thoughtful and thorough look at vaccine safety. We will examine:

- The science behind how vaccines are developed, tested, and monitored
- The systems in place to detect and report adverse reactions (such as VAERS and VSD)
- Common concerns about vaccine ingredients and how safety thresholds are determined
- Peer-reviewed studies and regulatory agency data that shed light on both real and perceived risks

We'll also discuss how regulatory bodies like the CDC, FDA, NIH, and WHO monitor vaccine safety and respond to concerns. Our goal is not to dismiss questions, but to explore them through the lens of credible evidence, sound science, open inquiry, and to better understand both the strengths and limitations of our current vaccine safety systems.

This exploration is essential for fostering public trust and making informed choices, particularly in a world where misinformation can spread quickly and medical decisions carry long-term consequences.

Let's start with safety studies (or the lack of them).

Do Vaccines Undergo Gold-Standard Safety Testing?

In medicine, *double-blind, placebo-controlled trials* are considered the gold standard for determining the safety and efficacy of new treatments. These studies involve giving one group the actual product and another group an inert placebo (such as saline), with neither the participants nor the researchers knowing who received what. This helps eliminate bias and isolate the true effects of the treatment. These trials usually continue for an extended period of time… several months to years in most cases.

However, when it comes to vaccines, especially those administered to infants and children, this standard is not applied in the same way.

Real-World Practices

When you hear the phrase "vaccine safety study," you might picture a rigorous, double-blind, years-long process where scientists carefully test a new vaccine against a completely inert placebo (like saline) and watch what happens over time. But in reality, that's not always how it works.

In many cases, the so-called "placebo" isn't actually a placebo at all. Instead of using something neutral like saline, they'll give the comparison group another vaccine. That's like testing whether a punch to the gut hurts by comparing it to a slap in the face. Sure, maybe one's less intense, but neither is exactly harmless.

And it doesn't stop there. Some of these studies are open-label or single-blind, which basically means someone in the process knows who's getting what. Either the person giving the shot, the person getting it, or both. That kind of defeats the whole purpose of a blind study, doesn't it?

Now toss in the fact that some vaccines are fast-tracked (especially under emergency or accelerated approval routes) and you've got even fewer hoops to jump through. Testing timelines can be shortened. Oversight gets a little looser. The urgency supposedly justifies the shortcuts.

And here's the kicker: in some of these trials, the safety data that ends up getting presented to the public is gathered from studies that last only a few days or weeks. Not months. Not years. Just long enough to see if someone has an immediate reaction, but not nearly long enough to detect delayed effects or long-term issues.

So when people say, "It's been tested for safety," it's worth asking, how was it tested, for how long, and what were they comparing it to? Because the devil, as always, is in the details.

So why is all this allowed? Why do vaccine studies often skip the true placebo or rush through short timelines?

Regulators usually say it's because it would be "unethical" to withhold a standard vaccine from the control group. In other words, they argue it's wrong not to vaccinate someone during a trial, even if the point of the trial is to see how safe or effective that vaccine really is.

And sure, on the surface, that might sound noble. But look a little closer and the logic starts to fall apart.

If we never test against an actual inert placebo, like saline, how can we possibly know what's causing what? How can we detect subtle or long-term side effects without a true baseline for comparison?

Are we really prioritizing public health... or just avoiding answers we might not want to hear?

And here's the uncomfortable part: most of these trials aren't being done on sick people. They're often being done on healthy children. Kids who aren't ill. Kids whose immune systems are already functioning well. So shouldn't that demand even *more* caution, not less?

One final question that doesn't get asked nearly enough: if something does go wrong—if that product causes harm—who exactly is held accountable? The answer to that, as you'll see in chapter 8, might be the most telling part of all.

Even mainstream scientists and health policy experts have raised their eyebrows about this.

A 2012 paper published in *Human & Experimental Toxicology* highlighted the lack of long-term, placebo-controlled safety studies in the childhood vaccine schedule[4].

The *Institute of Medicine* (now the National Academy of Medicine) in multiple reports has acknowledged the need for better research on cumulative vaccine exposure and safety outcomes over time[5].

A Double Standard in Drug Approval: Why Vaccines Are Treated Differently

In the realm of pharmaceuticals, rigorous testing is non-negotiable. Every drug, whether it's a common over-the-counter pain reliever or a complex chemotherapy agent, must pass through multiple phases of clinical trials before it can reach the public. These trials can span years, and for good reason: drug companies must prove not only effectiveness but also safety, especially over the long term.

To understand the depth of this system, consider a cancer patient whose prognosis is terminal. Even in this desperate situation, patients often cannot access experimental cancer drugs unless they are enrolled in tightly controlled trials or granted compassionate use exemptions, which are rare and difficult to obtain.

Why? Because these drugs have not yet been proven safe or effective, and regulators assert a duty to protect patients from potential harm, even when the alternative is death.

Yet, when it comes to vaccines, which are administered to healthy individuals, including infants and children, the ethical standards are often lost.

The Inert Placebo Dilemma: A Contradiction in Logic

Health agencies like the CDC, FDA, and WHO have frequently argued that using true saline placebos in vaccine trials would be unethical, because it would "withhold protection" from disease. But this rationale collapses under scrutiny:

- If withholding an unapproved product is unethical, then *all drug trials would be unethical.*

- If a treatment has not been proven to be safe or effective, how can it be assumed to be *protective at all*?
- Vaccines, like any other medical intervention, should *require proof* before assumption.

This ethical argument also contradicts standard practices in drug testing, where placebos are routine and even life-saving medications are withheld for the sake of clean data and patient safety.

Now here's where things get even more concerning. Vaccines are often studied without a true placebo. The control group might get another vaccine, or a shot filled with adjuvants (ingredients that aren't neutral at all). That kind of setup does a great job of blurring the data. If both groups experience side effects, it's harder to know where those effects are actually coming from.

These trials are also frequently done on relatively small groups of people. The follow-up period might only last a few weeks, maybe a couple months. Then, based on those limited studies, the product gets approved and rolled out to the public, sometimes even mandated. All this for a product that's going into the arms of newborns, children, pregnant women... some of the most vulnerable people in the population.

This would never fly in any other drug trial. But for vaccines, the rules seem to bend, break, or disappear entirely.

So let's take a closer look. Because when vaccines are approved without ever being tested against an inert substance, without a real placebo, any claims of safety are on shaky ground. And once you understand how these trials are actually run, it's hard not to question just how much we've been told is based on "settled science"... and how much is just carefully managed perception.

So let's explore examples of vaccines that were approved without undergoing true placebo-controlled trials, which means they were not tested against an inert substance like saline, but rather compared to another vaccine or adjuvant, often masking potential adverse effects. This practice stands in sharp contrast to standard pharmaceutical testing protocols and raises important questions about the validity of safety claims.

A Few of the Many Vaccines Approved Without True Placebo-Controlled Trials:

1. HPV Vaccine (Gardasil)
- **Approved**: 2006
- **Manufacturer**: Merck
- **Key Issue**: The placebo used in Gardasil trials was not inert saline, but rather the *aluminum adjuvant* (AAHS) also used in the vaccine.
- **Why it matters**: Aluminum is a known *immune-reactive substance*. By comparing Gardasil to a substance that already causes immune activation, it made adverse events appear similar between the groups, potentially obscuring the vaccine's true safety profile.
- **Quote from Merck's clinical protocol**: *"The placebo used in the control group was the vaccine carrier solution containing the same aluminum adjuvant."*

- **Implication**: The trial design may have underreported the rate of side effects, since the "placebo" could cause similar reactions.

2. Hepatitis B Vaccine
- **Approved:** Early 1980s
- **Placebo Comparison:** Some Hep B vaccines, especially early recombinant versions, were tested against *previous versions* or other vaccines.
- **No true placebo:** In many trials, there was *no inert saline group*. Instead, *"comparative studies"* were used between vaccine formulations or against older vaccines.
- **Administered to:** Newborns within 24 hours of birth, despite extremely low risk of exposure to hepatitis B for infants not born to infected mothers.
- **Clinical trials**: lasted only 5 days after dose.

3. Influenza Vaccines
- **Annual Updates:** Influenza vaccines are re-formulated and approved annually based on strain *prediction*.
- **No placebo trials:** Because each year's vaccine is "tweaked," they are approved under the assumption that they are "substantially equivalent" to prior versions, thus *bypassing the requirement for placebo-controlled trials altogether.*
- **Implication:** New formulations are *not subject to fresh long-term safety testing,* despite new combinations of antigens and adjuvants each year.

4. COVID-19 mRNA injections

- **Emergency Use Authorization (EUA):** Pfizer & Moderna received EUA in late 2020.
- **Early trials (Phase III):** Did initially include placebo groups (saline), but shortly after EUA was granted, placebo participants were offered the mRNA injection, *effectively ending long-term placebo comparison.*
- **Follow-up periods**: Were shortened. Original placebo-controlled design *was not completed* over the intended 2-year monitoring period.
- **Result:** We lack complete, long-term data comparing vaccinated vs. unvaccinated participants.

5. DTaP (Diphtheria, Tetanus, and Pertussis)
- **Approved:** 1990s, replacing whole-cell DTP
- **Trial Comparisons**: Often conducted against *other pertussis-containing vaccines*, not saline.
- **Concern:** Without a true placebo group, distinguishing side effects caused by the new formulation is difficult.

Why It Matters

True placebo-controlled trials are the **gold standard** of medical research. Without them, it's impossible to determine the **true baseline risk** of adverse events. This issue is especially pressing for vaccines, which are:

- Administered to healthy people
- Often *mandated* or required for access to education or employment

- Given repeatedly over a lifetime

This pattern of avoiding true placebos raises serious ethical and scientific concerns. It undermines trust, limits transparency, and *complicates the risk-benefit analysis* for both individuals and public health.

A profound contradiction lies at the heart of the public discourse on vaccine safety and advocacy. Those who raise concerns about vaccines or decline them are often derided for *"not following the science."* Yet, paradoxically, it is often the strongest proponents of widespread vaccination who depart from the gold standard of scientific inquiry. The scientific method demands rigorous, unbiased testing, including randomized, double-blind, true placebo-controlled trials, to establish both safety and efficacy. However, as we have seen, many vaccines are approved without ever undergoing such trials, or with comparisons to non-inert placebos that obscure real adverse effects.

When legitimate questions are raised about this departure from sound methodology, they are frequently dismissed, not answered. Ironically, this reveals that it is not the skeptics, but the

> **It is not the skeptics, but the most vocal advocates, who in many cases fail to uphold the foundational principles of science.**

most vocal advocates, who in many cases fail to uphold the foundational principles of science.

True scientific integrity does not fear scrutiny — it invites it.

"Trust the Experts." Who Are We to Question Them?

That's the phrase we've heard over and over again. Trust the experts. Don't question. Don't think too hard. Just follow the science.

But here's the problem: what happens when the "experts" don't follow the gold standard of science themselves? What happens when safety studies are rushed, sloppily designed, or missing entirely? Are we still supposed to nod our heads and go along with it?

The answer is no. Not blindly.

Real science evolves. What's considered expert opinion today might be completely overturned tomorrow when better data comes along. And that's not a flaw. That's actually how science is supposed to work. The problem starts when we treat it like dogma instead of a method.

Blind trust is not the same as informed trust. There's nothing wrong with respecting expertise, but it should come with questions, not obedience. You don't have to be a scientist to think critically. You just have to be willing to ask, *"Where's the evidence?"* and *"Who benefits from this recommendation?"*

Remember, science doesn't belong to the experts. It belongs to the process, (i.e. reproducible results, open debate, peer review, transparency) and the best scientists don't get offended when questioned. They welcome it. Because the moment we're not allowed to ask questions, it stops being science and starts being something else entirely.

So let's look at a few examples of what happens when we blindly trust the people in charge. Spoiler: it hasn't always gone well.

When Doctors Recommended Cigarettes: A Cautionary Tale of Expert Consensus

In the early-to-mid 20th century, cigarette smoking wasn't just socially acceptable, it was actively recommended by many in the medical community. Cigarette advertisements from the 1930s through the 1950s often featured physicians in white coats promoting their preferred cigarette brand. Slogans like *"More doctors smoke Camels than any other cigarette"* weren't just clever marketing, they reflected a cultural reality in which the medical establishment had not yet recognized, or publicly acknowledged, the health dangers of tobacco use.

At the time, the medical community lacked long-term epidemiological studies on smoking. The harmful effects, such as lung cancer, emphysema, and heart disease, often took decades to manifest.

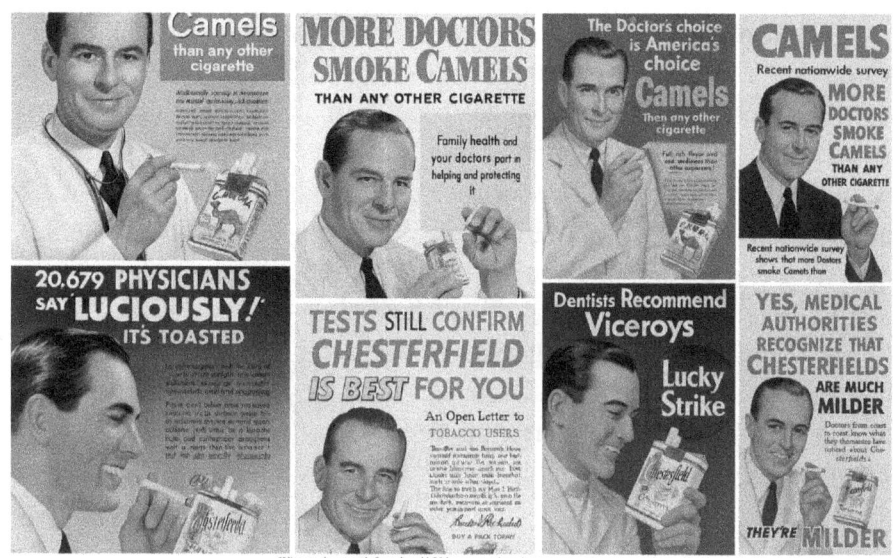

*Vintage cigarette ads from the mid-20th century, where doctors were used to promote tobacco. Used here under fair use for critical commentary.

Meanwhile, *tobacco companies funded research, influenced public opinion, and even supported medical associations financially.* Early concerns raised by independent researchers were often dismissed, ridiculed, or suppressed, further delaying public acknowledgment of the dangers.

It wasn't until the 1964 U.S. Surgeon General's report (decades after the initial rise in cigarette popularity) that a strong, official link was made between smoking and serious health problems. By then, smoking was deeply entrenched in global culture, and millions had become addicted under the impression that it was harmless or even beneficial.

What This Teaches Us.

The medical community is made up of humans who operate within cultural, financial, and political systems. While scientific knowledge progresses and eventually self-corrects, history shows that what is "expert consensus" at one time may not hold up under future scrutiny. The example of doctors once endorsing cigarettes illustrates the danger of blind trust, not in science itself, but in prematurely settled consensus and institutions that may have conflicting interests.

Therefore, questioning expert claims and demanding rigorous, independent science is not anti-science, it's how science evolves. Blind faith in any consensus without transparency, evidence, and accountability can lead to public health missteps with lasting consequences.

Is It Any Different Now?

If this all sounds familiar, it should. The tobacco industry once played from the same playbook that big pharma uses today: fund the research, shape the narrative, and buy the loyalty of medical associations. Doctors in white coats swore cigarettes were safe while industry-paid scientists cranked out reassuring studies. Now, swap out "cigarettes" for "vaccines" and it's déjà vu. The very companies that profit from today's vaccines are also the ones funding the safety studies, sponsoring the professional associations, and bankrolling the public messaging. If that doesn't set off alarm bells, it might be because the "smoke" is thicker this time around.

Artificial Sweeteners

Now let's talk about artificial sweeteners, those sugar substitutes that popped up over the last century and were once seen as miracle ingredients. But as we've seen, the story isn't quite so sweet.

Take saccharin, for example. It first hit the scene way back in the early 1900s. During sugar shortages, it became the go-to alternative… calorie-free and widely used. People loved it. But by the 1970s, things started to change. Studies on lab rats showed a link between saccharin and bladder cancer. That was enough for Congress to step in. Suddenly, saccharin had warning labels, and it landed on a government list of possible cancer-causing substances.

Then there's aspartame. You probably know it by brand names like NutraSweet or Equal. It got FDA approval in 1981 and quickly became the darling of the diet soda world. But it didn't take long for concerns to surface. People started reporting headaches, dizziness, even seizures after consuming it. And there's been a long-running debate about whether it affects the brain. Just recently, in 2023, the World Health Organization's cancer research arm (IARC) classified aspartame as "possibly carcinogenic to humans" because of studies showing a possible link to liver cancer. That raised a lot of eyebrows.

Sucralose (sold as Splenda) is another one that was thought to be completely safe when it came out in 1998. The belief was that it passed right through your system without causing harm. But newer research paints a different picture. Studies now suggest that sucralose might mess with your gut bacteria, affect how your body handles insulin, and even break down into harmful compounds when heated. In fact, a 2023 study published in *Toxicology and Environmental Health* found that sucralose can break down into a substance that may damage your DNA[31] — pretty serious stuff.

These examples show that expert consensus can shift, not because experts were malicious or incompetent, but because science is a process of discovery, self-correction, and refinement.

The Thalidomide Tragedy: When Expert Endorsement Led to a Global Health Crisis

In the late 1950s and early 1960s, thalidomide was marketed in nearly 50 countries as a safe, effective sedative and treatment for morning sickness in pregnant women. Developed by the German pharmaceutical company Chemie Grünenthal, the drug was widely prescribed and recommended by doctors across Europe, South America, and parts of Asia. Its safety profile was promoted heavily. Experts at the time assured the public it was non-toxic and well-tolerated, even in pregnant women.

However, the expert consensus was tragically and catastrophically wrong.

Thousands of babies were born with severe birth defects, primarily phocomelia, a condition where limbs are severely shortened or missing. In many cases, they appeared to have short flippers instead of arms and legs. It's estimated that more than 10,000 children across the world were affected. Some countries, like the United States, narrowly avoided widespread tragedy due to regulatory hesitation. Dr. Frances Kelsey of the U.S. Food and Drug Administration (FDA) famously refused to approve thalidomide without sufficient safety data, effectively preventing its mass distribution in the U.S.

At the time, few regulations required rigorous teratogenic (latin for "causing or producing monstrous development") testing for medications. Thalidomide passed what testing existed, and medical professionals trusted the limited data they were given, data that turned out to be incomplete and misleading. The disaster shocked the world and led to sweeping reforms in drug approval processes, including stricter requirements for safety testing and informed consent.

The thalidomide case reveals how dangerous it can be to rely solely on expert authority without transparency, independent verification, or comprehensive testing. It shows that well-intentioned professionals, when operating under faulty assumptions or *limited data*, can still contribute to massive harm. It also highlights the importance of regulatory vigilance and the value of dissent — Dr. Kelsey's refusal to approve the drug saved countless American lives.

This tragedy stands as a sobering reminder: expert consensus is not infallible. Public trust must be earned and sustained through rigorous, transparent science, not assumed by credential or position alone. Questioning medical and scientific recommendations is not a rejection of science but a necessary part of ensuring its integrity.

Mercury Amalgam Fillings: A Legacy of Trust That Is Being Reconsidered

For more than 150 years, mercury amalgam fillings have been a standard material used by dentists around the world to treat cavities.

These fillings, commonly referred to as "silver fillings," contain a mixture of metals (approximately *50% elemental mercury,* combined with silver, tin, and copper). For decades, dental associations and health regulatory agencies around the world, including the American Dental Association (ADA) and the U.S. Food and Drug Administration (FDA), insisted that mercury amalgam fillings were safe and effective.

Patients were rarely informed that their fillings contained mercury, a *well-documented neurotoxin,* and those who raised concerns were often dismissed as alarmist or anti-science. Dentists themselves were taught in dental school that amalgam posed no health threat, and most followed that guidance in good faith.

However, over time, growing evidence and evolving science began to challenge this expert consensus. Mercury vapor release studies have shown that amalgam fillings can release small amounts of mercury vapor, particularly when chewing, grinding teeth, or drinking hot liquids.

Bioaccumulation of mercury can accumulate in the body over time, and chronic low-level exposure has been linked to neurological, immunological, and renal issues.

Vulnerable populations of mercury amalgam fillings have been identified by health organizations to include certain groups including pregnant women, *children*, and people with mercury sensitivities.

In 2020, the FDA issued updated guidance about recommending mercury amalgam fillings.[6]

Many countries, including Sweden, Norway, and Denmark, have banned or severely restricted the use of mercury amalgam fillings altogether. Others are transitioning away from them in favor of composite resins and other mercury-free alternatives.

The mercury filling controversy underscores several key points:

- Expert consensus can shift as new evidence emerges.
- The absence of immediate, visible harm is not proof of safety, especially when dealing with substances like mercury that can cause subtle, long-term effects.
- Regulatory and professional assurances do not guarantee public safety, especially when economic or practical convenience is prioritized.

Despite years of reassurances from dental authorities, mercury fillings are now being scrutinized and phased out in many regions. Critics weren't wrong and the science caught up to their concerns.

The story of mercury amalgam dental fillings serves as a powerful reminder that public health guidance must be based on rigorous, transparent science, not merely professional tradition or authority. Just as with cigarettes, thalidomide, and artificial sweeteners, the history of mercury in dental care invites us to ask better questions, demand better answers, and never stop scrutinizing the claims of "settled science."

Drugs Once Approved, Then Withdrawn: A Pattern of Medical Reversal

The history of medicine is filled with examples of drugs that were enthusiastically embraced by the medical establishment, approved by regulators like the FDA, and widely prescribed, only to be later pulled from the market due to harmful or even deadly consequences. These cases expose the inherent fallibility of medical consensus, the limitations of pre-approval testing, and the systemic vulnerability to pharmaceutical industry influence.

Let's talk about some real-life examples that show how even FDA-approved drugs, sometimes wildly popular and doctor-recommended, turned out to be seriously dangerous.

Vioxx (Rofecoxib)

Vioxx hit the market in 1999 as a go-to treatment for arthritis and pain. It was supposed to be a safer alternative to other anti-inflammatories. But by 2004, it was pulled off the shelves. Why? Because post-market studies showed it *significantly* raised the risk of heart attacks and strokes.

Estimated 27,000 to 60,000 people may have died from cardiovascular complications.

Fen-Phen

Back in the 90s, Fen-Phen (a combo of fenfluramine and phentermine) was the weight-loss trend everyone was chasing. But it wasn't FDA-approved as a combo — and by 1997, it was pulled. Why? It was causing *serious* heart valve problems and rare lung diseases.

Thousands of lawsuits later, the manufacturer paid billions in settlements.
Lesson learned: Just because something's backed by "experts" doesn't make it safe long-term.

DES (Diethylstilbestrol)

Doctors prescribed DES starting in the 1940s to prevent miscarriages. It was given to millions of pregnant women. But by the 1970s, the truth came out: DES didn't prevent miscarriages, and worse, it caused rare cancers and fertility issues in the *daughters* of the women who took it.

This was one of the first clear cases of *multigenerational harm* from a drug.

Baycol (Cerivastatin)

Statins are a popular class of drugs, but Baycol turned out to be one of the more dangerous outliers. Approved in 1997, it was yanked by 2001 after it was linked to *rhabdomyolysis,* a serious muscle condition that can lead to kidney failure and even death. Over 100 people died before it was pulled.

Darvon/Darvocet (Propoxyphene)

These painkillers were on the market from 1957 to *2010* — more than 50 years. For decades, there were concerns about heart toxicity. But it wasn't until new data came in showing abnormal heart rhythms and sudden deaths that the FDA finally pulled them. Millions took it over half a century.

Lesson: Some drugs stay on the market long after red flags are raised... and the public pays the price.

Why This Matters

Each of these drugs passed expert review, clinical trials, and regulatory approval. Patients trusted their doctors. Doctors trusted the research. The research was often funded or influenced by pharmaceutical companies. When harm became undeniable, the damage was already done.

These examples echo a consistent truth:

"Consensus can be wrong. Approval is not a guarantee of safety. And experts, no matter how well-intentioned, can make grave mistakes."

Hormone Replacement Therapy (HRT)

For decades, Hormone Replacement Therapy (HRT) was widely promoted as a miracle treatment for postmenopausal women. Doctors prescribed it routinely to manage menopausal symptoms such as hot flashes and mood changes, but also for chronic disease prevention, including heart disease, osteoporosis, and even Alzheimer's.

Pharmaceutical companies marketed estrogen (often combined with progestin) aggressively under brands like Premarin and Prempro, and many doctors echoed the claim that HRT was essential for aging gracefully and staying healthy. The prevailing medical consensus, reinforced by expert panels and professional societies, was that HRT was not only safe, but beneficial for long-term use.

However, this consensus was overturned in 2002, when the Women's Health Initiative (WHI), a massive, government-funded, randomized controlled trial involving over 160,000 women, was halted early due to alarming findings.

What the WHI Revealed:

The Women's Health Initiative, launched by the NIH in the 1990s, sought to confirm the supposed benefits of HRT. Instead, it revealed significant risks, including:

- Increased risk of breast cancer
- Higher rates of stroke
- Greater incidence of heart attacks
- Higher rates of blood clots

The results shocked the medical world. Overnight, prescriptions for HRT plummeted, and countless women who had trusted their doctors were left confused and concerned.

The idea that HRT was a panacea for disease prevention had been *completely debunked*.

Key takeaways include:

- Widespread, expert-endorsed recommendations were based on observational studies, not randomized controlled trials.
- It took a large-scale, independent study to uncover the serious dangers previously unacknowledged.
- Millions of women were prescribed HRT under false pretenses, exposing them to unnecessary risks for years.

The HRT story is a sobering example of how medical "consensus" can be built on flawed or incomplete evidence. Trusted experts promoted HRT based on weak data, while critics who questioned its safety were marginalized. It took robust, unbiased science to correct the record, but by then considerable harm had been done.

The HRT reversal reminds us that challenging mainstream medical guidance isn't anti-science, it's *necessary* for scientific progress and patient safety. Just as with thalidomide, mercury amalgams, and smoking, the HRT debacle underscores the importance of not blindly trusting the experts, especially when large-scale pharmaceutical profits and widespread medical practice are at stake.

If this happened with all of the above examples, what current treatments might we be misunderstanding or misrepresenting, particularly those, like vaccines, that are promoted with similar certainty and trust in authority?

When it comes to vaccines, or any intervention promoted as "safe and effective," skepticism is not anti-science. It's pro-accountability.

The pattern of medical reversals demands vigilance and transparency, not blind obedience to authority.

History reminds us: "Following the science" must always include questioning the consensus, especially when lives are at stake. It also raises an important question for today's vaccination program:

What's In A Shot?

The absence of true randomized, double-blind, saline placebo-controlled trials in vaccine research creates a significant blind spot in our understanding of vaccine safety. Unlike other pharmaceuticals, which must meet strict safety standards through rigorous clinical testing, many vaccines are approved using comparison groups that receive other vaccines or adjuvant-containing solutions, rather than inert placebos. This makes it difficult to determine whether adverse effects are due to the vaccine itself or the *ingredients* used in both groups. Without a neutral baseline, the ability to identify risks is compromised.

This brings us to a critical concern: If vaccines are not tested against true placebos, then how can we accurately assess the safety of the *ingredients they contain*?

It is within this gap that the safety implications of vaccine components must be carefully examined.

Do you know what's in a vaccine? Most people don't. It's assumed by most, that the vaccines just contain a weak pathogen to stimulate immunity. Nothing could be further from the truth.

Imagine this scene: Jamie and Alex are sitting outside a café, sipping coffee after grocery shopping.

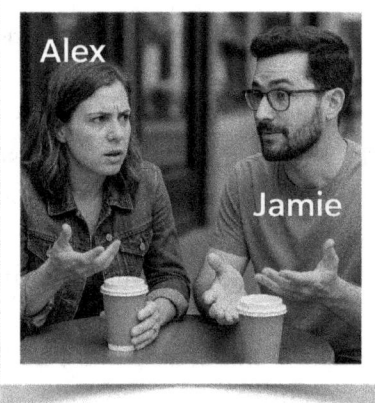

Jamie: You know, I've started reading food labels a lot more closely. It's crazy how much artificial stuff ends up in what we eat—preservatives, dyes, synthetic chemicals. I've cut out a bunch of it.
Alex: Yeah, me too. I stopped buying anything with artificial sweeteners or seed oils. If it has more than five ingredients I can't pronounce, I usually skip it.
Jamie: Exactly. That's why I started looking into what's in vaccines too.
Alex: (pauses and scowls) Wait… vaccines? You're not one of those *anti-vaxxers*, are you?
Jamie: (laughs) Seriously? You just said you won't *eat* something because of the ingredients. How's that different? I want to know what's being *injected* into me. Isn't that the same logic?
Alex: It's not the same. Vaccines are science. The experts say they save lives. Who are we to question the experts?!

Jamie: And food keeps us alive too, right? Don't "experts" tell us what's "safe" to put in our foods as well? But that doesn't mean we eat blindly. You reject junk food because of the additives. I reject certain vaccines because of additives like aluminum, polysorbate 80, and formaldehyde. So... does that make you an *anti-fooder*?
Alex: (chuckles awkwardly) That's not a real thing.
Jamie: Neither is "anti-vaxxer" in the way people use it. It's a defamatory label to shut down questions. I'm not anti-anything... I'm pro-information. Same as you when you read a food label.
Alex: (sighs) I guess when you put it like that...
Jamie: Look, we're not saying *no*, we're saying *know*. Just like food, vaccines deserve transparency. People should be allowed to ask questions without being ridiculed.

Vaccine Ingredients

Now that we've highlighted the double standard in how society views ingredient awareness (accepting scrutiny in food but often dismissing it in vaccines), we turn our focus to a detailed exploration of what vaccines actually contain.

Understanding the ingredients is not a fringe concern but a matter of informed consent and personal health responsibility. Just as reading food labels empowers individuals to make choices aligned with their values and health needs, knowing the components of vaccines allows for the same level of scrutiny.

In the following section, we will examine, one by one, the ingredients commonly found in vaccines, such as adjuvants, preservatives, stabilizers, and residuals from the manufacturing process. I'll use data and documentation provided by respected sources, including the CDC, FDA, WHO, NIH, EPA, and vaccine manufacturer inserts. This analysis will not only identify each ingredient but also explain its function and raise important questions about its safety, especially when injected into the body repeatedly over time.

Mercury (Thimerosal/Thiomersal)

Remember those days when thermometers were filled with that shiny, silvery liquid... mercury? It seemed like magic, didn't it? Kids would find endless fascination in the way the little beads of mercury would glide and split apart when a thermometer broke. It felt so unique, almost like a science experiment right on your kitchen floor! But as we all know now, that enchanting liquid came with a hefty warning label.

Parents were soon alerted to the dangers of mercury, explaining how easily our bodies could absorb it and the serious health consequences that could follow. *"Don't play with mercury!"*

It's funny how something so captivating turned out to be so perilous, transforming our innocent play into a health hazard. Why? Because for decades, mercury has been an ingredient in many vaccines!

Before we discuss mercury in vaccines, it is important to mention:

In the summer of 2025, something amazing happened. Something unexpected. Something surprisingly, yet profoundly, unforeseen. In June of that year, the CDC Advisory Committee on

Immunization Practices, following a recommendation by Robert F. Kennedy, Jr., the Secretary of the US Department of Health and Human Services, voted to recommend a full ban on mercury-containing preservatives in all vaccines. Just a month later, in July 2025, Kennedy formally approved this recommendation, aligning U.S. vaccine policies with those of other developed nations.

While this decision represents a significant step forward, the conversation surrounding mercury in vaccines remains far from over. For decades, mercury has been injected into pregnant women, children, and adults, often without their knowledge or consent. The millions of people who have unknowingly been subjected to this toxic substance must now confront the long-term effects and the potential ramifications for their health.

Moreover, though the ban recommended by Kennedy's HHS is a crucial development, it is important to note that this is just the beginning. As of the publication of this book, the removal of mercury from vaccines has not yet been fully implemented by the vaccine manufacturers. And given the political climate, it is not only possible but highly plausible that future administrations—motivated by financial incentives—may reverse this policy, potentially allowing mercury to re-enter vaccines.

Furthermore, as of this writing, global organizations such as the World Health Organization (WHO) and GAVI, the Global Vaccine Alliance, continue to recommend mercury-containing vaccines for hundreds of millions of children in underdeveloped countries. This raises critical questions about the future of mercury in vaccines and the ongoing risks for those who will continue to be subjected to them.

For all these reasons, the discussion on mercury in vaccines is far from over. It is essential to understand the full scope of its impact—both past and future—on individuals who have already been affected, those who will be, and the broader implications should mercury find its way back into vaccine formulations.

Now Let's Talk About Thimerosal

You might've heard people mention *thimerosal* when talking about vaccines, especially when concerns come up about mercury. So what is it, really? And is it something to worry about?

Thimerosal (also spelled thiomersal) is an organomercury compound that contains approximately 49.6% *mercury* by weight. It has been used as a preservative in some vaccines, especially multi-dose vials since the 1930s. It was added to prevent bacteria and fungi from growing in vaccine vials, especially those that were used for multiple doses.

Now, the word *mercury* tends to raise red flags… as it should!

There are different types of mercury. The type in thimerosal is called *ethylmercury*, while another form is called *methylmercury* (the type found in some fish and industrial pollutants). They're processed differently in the body but *both have risks.*

Let's be very clear about one thing… mercury, *in any form*, is toxic to the human body. Proponents of vaccine safety are famous for claiming that ethylmercury is safe as opposed to methylmercury.

However, both are forms of mercury, and both are toxic (don't play with mercury).

Mercury Is A Neurotoxin

Mercury, in all its forms, is known to be toxic to the nervous system. Ethylmercury, an organic mercury compound, can accumulate in the brain and disrupt normal neurological function, as well as renal toxicity causing kidney failure.[1]

How Is It Processed in the Body?

Ethylmercury is metabolized in the body into inorganic mercury. Inorganic mercury is indisputably toxic! According to the National Institutes of Health (NIH):

> *"Upon administration, ethylmercury quickly dissociates from thiosalicylic acid and binds to blood or other tissue. The toxicological profile of ethylmercury from thimerosal is thought to be **similar** to that of ethylmercury from other sources (Magos, 2001b; Suzuki et al., 1963, 1973).*
>
> *"**Mercury is clearly neurotoxic and nephrotoxic**. Organic mercury forms of interest, ethyl- and methylmercury, are metabolized to mercuric mercury. The effects of mercuric mercury are greatest in the **kidneys**, whereas the effects of organic mercury are greatest in the **central and peripheral nervous systems** (Aschner and Aschner, 1990). Generally, mercury is thought to induce cytotoxicity through inhibition of protein synthesis and cellular enzyme-mediated reactions, resulting in structural changes of cells, interference with cellular metabolism, and inhibition of cell migration (Clarkson, 1972). More specifically, mercuric mercury exposure can cause **acute renal failure and toxicity**, characterized by proteinuria, oliguria, and hematuria. Case studies have also reported congested medulla, pale and swollen cortex, extensive necrosis, and degeneration of tubular epithelium (ATSDR, 1999). Similar*

> *measures of toxicity such as necrosis of proximal tubules, proteinuria, and general renal nephropathy have been demonstrated in animal studies (ATSDR, 1999)."[1]* (emphasis mine)

And pay attention to this one:

> *"Many features of the toxicity of ethylmercury are thought likely to be **qualitatively similar to those of methylmercury** (Ball et al., 2001)[1]."* (emphasis mine)

To put it simply, according to the NIH, both types of mercury have similar destructive effects on the body.

Even in light of this known data, some of the biggest public health agencies, like the CDC, FDA, World Health Organization (WHO), and Institute of Medicine (IOM), continue to claim that they can find no credible evidence or connection that thimerosal in vaccines causes harm.

Why? This rationale is a result of **inductive** reasoning:

Observation: There is no evidence that thimerosal causes harm.
Conclusion: Since there is no connection, thimerosal is safe.

Whereas the logical, **deductive** mind can *easily* make the obvious connection:

Premise 1: Mercury is toxic to the central and peripheral nervous system and kidneys.[1]

Premise 2: According to the substantial data, like that found in the NIH database, ethylmercury is qualitatively similar to methylmercury.[1]
Premise 3: Thimerosal contains ethylmercury.
Conclusion: Thimerosal is toxic to the human body.

Another argument that public health agencies like the CDC, FDA, and WHO maintain is that these substances are included in extremely small, regulated amounts that are far below toxic thresholds.

But what about infants and children?

- Most safety data is based on adult exposures.
- Children, especially infants with immature organs and developing immune systems, respond differently to cumulative exposure.
- Dosing isn't always proportionally scaled to weight or body mass, which would be standard in other pharmacological practices.

This raises valid questions about *cumulative exposure* to biologically active or toxic compounds of 70+ doses of vaccines over childhood.

Keeping in mind that the NIH considers ethylmercury *qualitatively similar* to methylmercury, let's do some simple math:

- The EPA considers *acceptable* amounts of methylmercury = 5.8 microns (mcg) per liter of blood
- Therefore, (even though we know that *no* amount of mercury is actually safe) the EPA considers 5.8 mcg/liter as *"safe"* for *adults*.

- The average adult body contains approximately 5 liters of blood
- Therefore, 5.8 mcg of mercury x 5 liters of blood = 29 mcg *"safe"* for *adults*.
- The average newborn's body (8lbs) contains 270ml of blood (0.27 liters).
- Therefore according to the FDA, 5.8 mcg x 0.27 = 1.57 mcg "safe" for babies.
- According to the FDA: A vaccine containing thimerosal contains 25 micrograms of mercury *per dose*.[2]

25 mcg of mercury is almost *40 times higher* than the FDA acceptable amounts for babies... per dose!
[for age specific body weight calculations use 75ml blood/kg of body weight to know what is "considered safe" for your child]

Mercury and Neurological Consequences

Okay, so here's something pretty fascinating... and more than a little unsettling. Researchers at the University of Calgary's Faculty of Medicine did a study[3] that gave us one of the clearest looks yet at how mercury affects the brain... and they actually caught it *on camera*. Seriously.

They used *live neuron tissue cultures,* basically, brain cells growing in a dish, and watched what happened when they exposed those developing neurons to mercury ions. What they saw was pretty dramatic. The neurons were dying right in front of their eyes. Shriveling back into themselves like the legs of the Wicked Witch of the East!

The mercury ions latched onto these little proteins called *tubulin*. Tubulin's job is to help build the "skeleton" of a neuron. Think of it like scaffolding that gives the cell its shape and helps it grow properly. But when mercury binds to tubulin, it can't do its job. So the scaffolding collapses. The neuron literally falls apart, including the growth cone, which is kind of like the "steering wheel" that helps the neuron connect with others.

As a result, the neuron doesn't just stop growing. it starts *breaking down*, and researchers even saw the formation of tangled proteins, which look very similar to the ones found in brains with Alzheimer's disease.

So why does this matter? Well, this study gave scientists visual, undeniable proof that mercury can directly damage brain cells, especially while they're still developing. It also adds weight to the theory that mercury exposure might be linked to neurodegenerative diseases. The damage they saw looked a *lot like* the same kind of damage found in the brains of people with Alzheimer's disease, specifically in about 80% of Alzheimer's cases!

Long story short: this is one of those studies that makes you think twice about mercury exposure, especially in kids when the brain is still wiring itself up.

Now, lets walk through to the *deductive* conclusion that connects the University of Calgary's mercury neuron degeneration research to vaccine-related mercury exposure, particularly thimerosal:

Premise 1: What the Calgary Research Showed

The University of Calgary researchers visually documented how mercury ions (Hg^{2+}) destroy neurons. In the video and associated study, they observed:
- Mercury binds to tubulin, a protein needed to build the scaffolding of neurons.
- This binding prevents microtubule formation, which is essential for neuron structure and transport of nutrients.
- As a result, the neuron collapses, and the growth cone retracts — a hallmark of *neurodegeneration*.
- These changes closely resembled what's seen in Alzheimer's disease brains.

This was powerful because it was *direct visual evidence* of how even very small amounts of mercury can have destructive effects on brain cells.

Premise 2: What Thimerosal Is
- Thimerosal is a *mercury-based preservative* (about 49.6% ethylmercury by weight) used in some vaccines and multi-dose vials to prevent bacterial contamination.
- Ethylmercury (in thimerosal) is qualitatively similar to methylmercury[1], and both are neurotoxic[1], especially to developing brains.
- The CDC and FDA have acknowledged that mercury exposure should be minimized, especially in infants and pregnant women.

Premise 3: The Connection
1. Visual proof of mercury's harm to neurons (Calgary study) shows how low levels of mercury can be neurotoxic, even

without full-body exposure. Just localized neuron contact is enough.
2. Thimerosal breaks down into ethylmercury, which crosses the blood-brain barrier and can accumulate in brain tissue.
3. Although ethylmercury is eliminated faster than methylmercury, it still enters the brain, and its exact long-term neurodevelopmental impact is still debated, especially with repeated dosing in early childhood.
4. Infants and fetuses have developing brains, which are more vulnerable to mercury's effects, which is exactly what the Calgary researchers were modeling.

Conclusion:
- Even though the Calgary neuron research wasn't specifically looking at thimerosal, it raises legitimate concerns about any source of mercury exposure, including thimerosal in vaccines, especially during critical periods of brain development.

To be fair, thimerosal was removed or reduced from most childhood vaccines in the U.S. and other countries starting in 1999, marking a significant shift in vaccine policy after decades of use. As of now, no U.S. childhood vaccines on the routine immunization schedule contain thimerosal. However, thimerosal has been injected into children and adults for generations, and the bioaccumulation of mercury has been building up for decades. Even today, millions of people, particularly in underdeveloped countries, continue to be exposed to this toxic substance. While the recent recommendation in 2025 from Robert F. Kennedy, Jr. and the U.S. Department of Health and Human Services to ban mercury-containing preservatives in vaccines is a positive step forward, the impact of past exposures cannot be ignored. Moreover, with the global vaccine recommendations from organizations like the WHO and GAVI continuing to include mercury-containing vaccines for children, the threat of mercury's reintroduction in vaccine formulations remains a very real concern for both current and future generations.

Aluminum

Yep, it's true. Aluminum is used in a bunch of vaccines, not as a preservative, but as something called an **adjuvant**.

You'll find aluminum in vaccines like DTaP, hepatitis A and B, HPV, and a few others.

But... Isn't Aluminum Bad for You?

You know, aluminum isn't just some harmless metal, it's actually a known neurotoxin. The National Institutes of Health (NIH) even says that aluminum can mess with *over 200 different biological processes* in the body, and it's especially harmful to the brain and nervous system. They've linked aluminum exposure to serious brain disorders like Alzheimer's, Parkinson's, multiple sclerosis, and even a condition called dialysis encephalopathy, basically a form of brain dysfunction caused by metal buildup in people on dialysis.

In other words, scientists are pretty clear: aluminum has real potential to harm the brain, especially when it builds up over time. So when people ask questions about why aluminum is in vaccines, or how it might affect developing brains, they're not being paranoid. They're pointing to real science that says aluminum isn't something to take lightly.

So here's where it gets interesting… and honestly, a little concerning for some people. The aluminum we just talked about, the one that's considered a neurotoxin and has been linked to brain-related diseases, is actually used in some vaccines as an adjuvant. That's a fancy word for an ingredient added to vaccines to stimulate your immune system so it reacts more strongly to the shot.

Now, here's the thing: this isn't the kind of aluminum you'd find in foil or soda cans. In vaccines, it's usually in the form of compounds like aluminum hydroxide or aluminum phosphate. These forms are *supposed* to be safe in small amounts, and the official line from public health agencies like the CDC and FDA is that they've been used for decades with no proven harm (inductive reasoning).

But some scientists and doctors have raised concerns, especially when it comes to babies and young kids. Why? Because their immune systems and brains are still developing, and injecting a neurotoxic metal, even in tiny amounts, directly into the body might carry different risks than when it's ingested or exposed through the environment. A few animal studies have suggested that repeated exposure to aluminum adjuvants could potentially lead to immune system problems or even neurological effects.

So when people ask questions like: "Why is aluminum in vaccines?" or, "Is it possible this could affect kids over time?", they're not rejecting science. They're actually paying attention to it. They're looking at what we already know about aluminum, and asking whether we've fully explored the long-term effects when it's injected into the body, especially in a schedule that includes multiple vaccines in a short period of time, and then continue throughout childhood and adulthood (deductive reasoning).

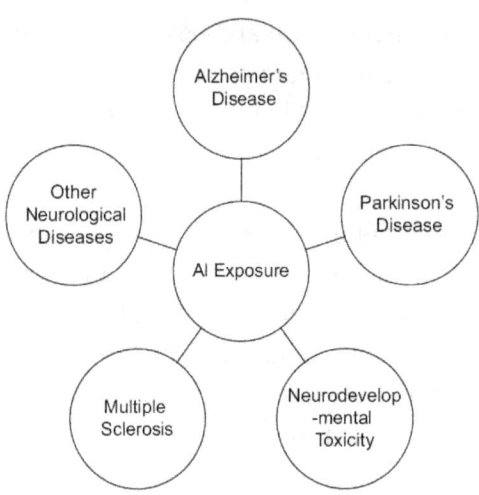

Aluminum is widely recognized in scientific literature as a neurotoxin with potential links to multiple neurological disorders. In a 2011 review published in the *International Journal of Alzheimer's Disease*[7], researchers Kawahara and Kato-Negishi explored how aluminum may contribute to the progression of Alzheimer's disease by disrupting neural function and exacerbating amyloid plaque formation.

Additional studies have noted its association with dialysis encephalopathy, ALS, and Parkinsonism-dementia syndromes observed in regions like the Kii Peninsula in Japan and Guam. Toxicologist Robert A. Yokel's earlier review also documented how aluminum can accumulate in the brain and affect its structure and function[8,10]. These findings have prompted concern about aluminum's role in long-term neurological health, especially with continued environmental and medical exposure.

So, how much aluminum is actually okay for humans?

The short answer is... none! It really depends however, on how you're exposed to it, whether you're eating it, drinking it, or getting it injected through something like a vaccine or IV.

Aluminum from Food and Water (Ingested)

For most people, the main way we're exposed to aluminum is through food. It's in fish, processed cheese, baking powder, some food colorings, even in our drinking water in small amounts.

- The FDA says bottled water can have up to 0.1 to 0.3 milligrams (mg) of aluminum per liter.[12,14]
- And the World Health Organization (WHO) has a guideline that says it's okay to consume about 2 mg of aluminum per kilogram of your body weight per week.[14] So, if you weigh around 150 pounds (about 70 kg), that would be up to 140 mg per week, or about 20 mg per day, mostly from food.[13]

That might sound like a lot, but your digestive system doesn't absorb much aluminum. Most of it just passes through without doing any harm.

Aluminum from Injections (Like Vaccines or IVs)

This is where it gets more complicated. When aluminum is injected, it bypasses your digestive system and goes straight into your body's tissues. That means your body absorbs it much more directly.

- The FDA allows up to 850 micrograms (which is 0.85 mg) of aluminum per vaccine dose.[14]
- This limit was set based on older safety data, not necessarily on the latest research about how aluminum behaves in the body, especially in babies.

People with kidney problems, or very young babies whose kidneys aren't fully developed, can have a hard time clearing aluminum from their system. Over time, if aluminum builds up, it can affect the brain and bones, this has actually been seen in people on long-term dialysis who were exposed to aluminum.

So, while small amounts of aluminum in food or water are generally "considered *safe*", we start to ask bigger questions when it comes to repeated injections, especially in infants, or in people with health conditions that make it hard to remove aluminum from the body.

The Aluminum Safety Limit Paradox

You know what's kind of strange? The "safe" limits for aluminum exposure, especially in vaccines, were mostly based on full-grown adults. Not babies. Not toddlers. Just healthy, average-sized adults.

And that's a big deal, because babies obviously aren't just mini adults. They have tiny bodies, developing brains, and kidneys that aren't fully ready to filter out stuff like aluminum. Yet, they're often

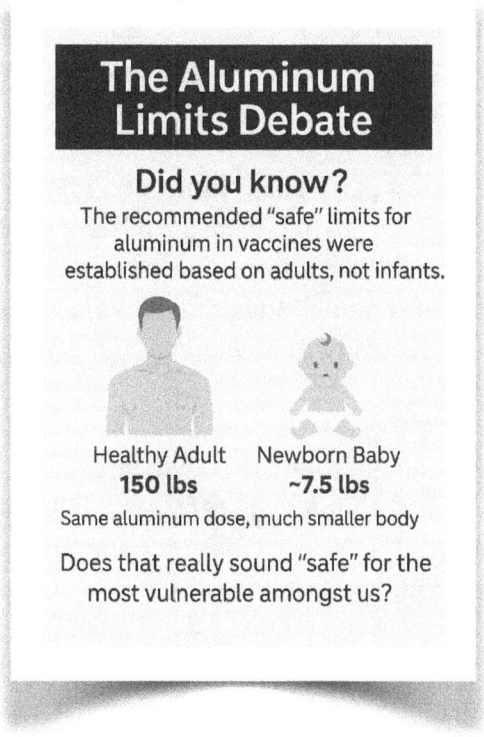

given the *same amount of aluminum per vaccine dose as an adult* would be, repetitively, throughout childhood!

Think about it this way: a healthy adult weighs around 150 pounds. A newborn? Maybe 7 or 8 pounds. So when a baby gets a shot with 225 or even 850 micrograms of aluminum, which is technically within the *"safe"* limit, they're getting a much *higher dose per pound of body weight* than an adult ever would.

That's kind of like giving a toddler a full adult dose of caffeine and saying, "It's fine, this is safe for a grown-up." Except aluminum is *much more dangerous*.

And the weirdest part? These limits don't really get adjusted downward for babies. It's not like there's a different standard for infants or kids. We just assume that it's fine, even though there are studies showing that aluminum can build up in tissues and affect things like brain development, especially in premature infants or babies with underdeveloped kidneys.

This raises valid questions about whether these limits on aluminum in infants and children are safe, especially those who receive multiple aluminum-containing vaccines on a single day and over the course of the entire childhood vaccine schedule!

Combine the neurotoxic findings of aluminum with the neurotoxicity of mercury and we can easily begin to deduce why long term neurological disorders like Autism, Parkinson's, Alzheimer's, Multiple Sclerosis, etc. have been on the rise… especially in an eerily similar path as the increase in the vaccine schedule (which we'll discuss later in the chapter).

Formaldehyde

So, let's say someone told you, "Hey, we're going to inject a tiny amount of formaldehyde into your child." You'd probably blink a few times and say, "Wait... isn't that the stuff they use to preserve dead bodies?" And you'd be right. Formaldehyde *is* used in embalming fluid. It's also classified as a known human carcinogen by major health agencies like the International Agency for Research on Cancer (IARC)[15]. Not exactly the kind of thing you'd expect to find in something meant to *keep you healthy*, right?

But here's the twist: formaldehyde is also a common ingredient in vaccines. Why? Because it's used during the manufacturing process to inactivate viruses or detoxify bacterial toxins. The idea is that it helps make the vaccine safer by neutralizing the parts that could cause illness, and most of the formaldehyde is removed before the final product ever reaches the needle.

Health authorities argue that the amount left behind is *extremely* small, usually less than what's naturally found in your own bloodstream. So they say: "Hey, don't worry, this little bit is totally safe." Yep, just like the health authorities who said smoking was safe, thalidomide was safe, mercury fillings were safe, etc.

Here's where things get... kind of ironic. The same substance that comes with hazard warnings in high school chemistry labs, and is tightly regulated in food, cosmetics, and furniture, is somehow "not a problem" when it's injected into a baby?

That's where a lot of people scratch their heads. Especially when it comes to kids, whose immune and detox systems are *still developing*. We worry about food dyes, plastic containers, and secondhand smoke, but we're totally okay with injecting trace embalming chemicals *as long as it's in a vaccine*?!

"Just a Little Extra Ingredient"

Imagine this Scene: Late afternoon. A cozy kitchen. Sunlight pours through the windows. A mother stands at the counter, pulling a tray of fresh brownies from the oven. The smell is heavenly.

Enter Jake (age 9) and Lily (age 7), messy from playing outside.

Jake: *(sniffing the air)*
Mmm... Mom, what *is* that smell?

Lily:
Are you baking brownies?! Please tell me those are brownies!

Mom: *(smiling)*
You two have good noses! Yep! Fresh out of the oven. I made a big pan just for us.

Jake: *(grinning)*
Can we have one *now*?

Mom:
Of course! But first, I want to tell you what's in them. Just so you know.

Lily: *(shrugging)*
Okay, but we already know. Flour, sugar, chocolate…

Mom:
Yep, all of that. Flour, sugar, cocoa, eggs, a bit of vanilla… and just a *tiny* bit of doggie poop.

Jake and Lily: *(both freeze)*
WHAT?!

Lily: *(wide-eyed)*
Dog poop?! Are you serious?

Mom: *(calmly)*
Just a teensy bit. You won't smell it. You won't taste it. And baking kills all the germs, so it's totally safe.

Jake: *(making a face)*
But… it's POOP!

Lily: *(gagging)*
Ewwww! I don't want poop brownies!

Mom:
But you wouldn't even *know* if I hadn't told you. Just a little bit. Practically nothing.

Jake: *(backing away)*
That's still gross. No way!

Lily: *(running out)*
I'm not eating those!

Mom: *(calling after them)*
Suit yourselves!

(She chuckles softly, looking at the untouched brownies.)

What Does This Have to Do With Vaccines?

This scene illustrates a paradox many people wrestle with when it comes to toxic ingredients in vaccines.

Health authorities often reassure the public that substances like aluminum, formaldehyde, or mercury-based preservatives are only present in vaccines in *very small amounts*, so small that they're considered safe.

But here's the catch:

- The kids reject the brownies not because the amount of poop is large, but because they understand that *any* amount of something known to be toxic or gross *matters,* especially when it's going *into* their bodies.

- The argument from health authorities is that dose makes the poison. That doesn't change how people feel when they learn what's inside. Poison *is* poison, especially when the ingredients involve substances that are toxic in any other context.

- Just like the brownies, you wouldn't know what's in the vaccine unless someone told you. The smell, the look, the "taste", all seem harmless. But the presence of something questionable, even in small doses, *can and does change perception.*

This story doesn't claim vaccines are brownies with poop in them. It raises a powerful point about transparency, consent, and trust, and how much people value knowing *exactly* what's going into their bodies or their children's bodies, no matter how small the dose.

It raises a fair question: Shouldn't we at least ask more questions about the long-term effects of introducing toxins like formaldehyde this way? Especially in combination with other toxic ingredients like aluminum and mercury for repeated doses throughout childhood?

So, while the experts assure us it's safe in small amounts, the average person might reasonably wonder: If it's too dangerous to put in baby shampoo, why is it okay in a shot?

Phenol/Phenoxyethanol

Alright, let's talk about another vaccine ingredient that tends to raise some eyebrows... *phenol* (or its more modern counterpart, *phenoxyethanol*). Now, most people haven't heard of these unless they're deep-diving into ingredient lists, but both are used in vaccines as preservatives to help keep the formula stable and free from contamination.

Here's where it gets interesting: phenol is actually classified as *toxic*. It's used in things like disinfectants, antiseptics, and even some industrial products. Phenoxyethanol, often seen as a "safer" alternative, is also found in cosmetics and personal care items, but with clear warnings not to use it on *broken skin* or in large amounts, *especially for infants.*

So here's the question that naturally follows: if these substances require caution in cosmetics and household products, how are we justifying their use in something as sensitive as a childhood vaccine, especially when these doses are injected and often given repeatedly throughout childhood (and into adulthood), sometimes in the same visit? And even if the amounts are *"small,"* does that automatically make them safe for a still-developing baby's system?

It's about *logic* and informed questioning. If we're careful about what we put *on* a child's skin, shouldn't we be just as cautious about what we're injecting *into* their body? Let's dig a little deeper, because that's where the conversation around phenoxyethanol really starts to pick up.

The FDA allows it in vaccines in small amounts, typically less than 1%, and regulators often say that at these levels, it's "generally recognized as safe." But here's the catch, most of that safety data is once again... based on *adult exposure*, not the cumulative impact on infants and toddlers receiving dozens of shots throughout early childhood.

What's more, phenoxyethanol comes with known side effects when overexposed. Things like skin irritation, nervous system suppression, and even organ damage in severe cases. In fact, the European Chemicals Agency (ECHA) classifies it as harmful if swallowed, and warns it may cause damage to organs through prolonged or repeated exposure. And interestingly, the manufacturer of one phenoxyethanol-containing product for babies once recalled it because it caused vomiting and diarrhea in infants... through *topical* use!

So again, we run into the same kind of paradox we've talked about with other ingredients: if something is harmful at higher doses, or with repeated exposure, and especially risky for babies externally, how can they say it's safe when injected directly into a developing child's body?

Now here's where things get even more curious. Did you know that phenol, (yes, the same compound used in some vaccines) was *once used as antifreeze*? Sounds strange, right? But it's true. Phenol was historically used in antifreeze formulations until manufacturers realized something concerning: it was *too corrosive* for the machinery. It literally damaged the parts it was supposed to protect.

Now pause for a moment and think about that. If a chemical is too harsh for metal and rubber, how does it make sense to inject it into developing human bodies... especially babies?

And it's not just a historical anecdote — the CDC itself still has some strong words about phenol. According to their official guidance:

> *"Phenol denatures proteins and generally acts as a protoplasmic poison. Phenol may also cause peripheral nerve damage (i.e., demyelination of axons). Systemic poisoning can occur after inhalation, skin contact, eye contact, or ingestion... Damage to the nervous system is the primary cause of death from phenol poisoning."*

That's not an obscure source... that's straight from the CDC. They even note that symptoms may not show up for up to 18 hours after exposure, which raises serious questions about how we monitor and detect delayed effects.

And here's where the conversation circles back to kids. The CDC *also* acknowledges that:

> *"Children do not always respond to chemicals in the same way that adults do. Different protocols for managing their care may be needed."*

Exactly. If children's bodies process chemicals differently (and more vulnerably) how are we accounting for that when these substances are included in the vaccine schedule that begins as early as the first day of life?

Again, this isn't about fear-mongering. It's about common sense. If phenol was too harsh for machines, and if it's recognized as a neurotoxic threat with delayed effects, and if children process toxins differently... doesn't it make sense to at least *question* its use in something as critical as childhood vaccines?

It's not just a scientific question, it's a moral one. Shouldn't the burden of proof for safety be *higher*, not lower, when it comes to our most vulnerable?

These are the kinds of questions that deserve open dialogue, not censorship, not dismissal, but serious, respectful discussion.

Alright, let's dig a little deeper into phenol and its close cousin phenoxyethanol, and the effects they can have on our bodies, especially when exposure is through injection, as is the case with certain vaccines.

According to the CDC, phenol isn't just some mild chemical that quietly slips through your system unnoticed. In fact, it can seriously impact multiple major systems in the body.

Shouldn't the burden of proof for safety be *higher*, not lower, when it comes to our most vulnerable?

Let's break it down and show what effects it can have on the different systems:

Central Nervous System (CNS):

Phenol exposure can start off with what seems like mild symptoms. Things like nausea, sweating, dizziness, or a ringing in your ears. But in more serious cases, it escalates fast. We're talking seizures, loss of consciousness, coma, and even death. What's particularly troubling is that these effects might not hit right away. Symptoms can be *delayed up to 18 hours*. That makes it incredibly difficult to link cause and effect.

Cardiovascular System:

Phenol can also wreak havoc on your heart and blood pressure. Initially, it might cause a spike in blood pressure, but that's often followed by a sharp drop, leading to severe low blood pressure, shock, irregular heartbeats, or dangerously slow heart rates. These aren't rare side effects. They've been documented, even with *skin* exposure.

Blood and Kidneys:

Phenol has also been linked to *renal failure,* (complete shutdown of the kidneys) in cases of acute poisoning. Tests have shown protein in the urine, weird discoloration (think green or brown), and other clear signs of kidney distress. On the blood side, phenol can damage the blood-forming organs. It also raises concerns for *methemoglobinemia,* especially in infants under one year old. This condition reduces the blood's ability to carry oxygen, and since babies already have lower hemoglobin levels than adults, that risk goes up even more.

Skin Exposure:

And this one's wild! If more than 60 square inches of your skin is exposed to phenol, there is a risk of *imminent death!* That's just a small area, not even half the size of a typical adult back. So, if it's *that toxic on your skin,* how does it make sense to *inject* it into infants?

Let's keep this conversation rolling, because the more we dig into phenol and phenoxyethanol, the more the questions pile up.

We've talked about the *acute* dangers, things like seizures, kidney failure, and serious cardiac issues that can happen after just a single significant exposure. But what about *chronic exposure*? What happens when small amounts are introduced over and over again, say during a childhood vaccine schedule?

Here's where it gets seriously concerning.

Potential Long-Term Effects (Sequelae)

Phenol isn't just dangerous in the short term. When someone is exposed acutely (even once) it can leave *lasting damage.* We're talking:

- **Chronic nerve damage** (once nerves are damaged, they don't always regenerate).
- **Chemical burns** that can cause ongoing skin or eye issues.
- If ingested? It can cause **esophageal narrowing,** basically a permanent narrowing of the tube you swallow through. As well as lasting **heart and kidney damage.**

That's a big deal, and now imagine if someone is exposed to it *repeatedly.*

Chronic Exposure (Over Time)

According to workplace studies, where employees are exposed to low levels of phenol repeatedly, some pretty serious trends have been documented:

- **Kidney damage** (inflammation, swelling, degenerative changes in key kidney structures).
- **Liver problems**, pigment changes in the skin.
- And notably, increased risk of coronary artery disease and poor blood supply to the heart.

Now let's stop and think: these were *adults*, exposed primarily through *skin contact or inhalation*. That's still pretty concerning. But in the context of vaccines, this chemical is *injected!* A much more direct route into the body.

And here's the part that should really make us think:

"Chronic exposure may be more serious for children because of their potential longer latency period." - CDC

That means the effects might not show up right away, but over time, as their systems develop, the consequences can be more significant.

How Does This Relate to Vaccines?

Vaccines are often administered *repeatedly,* sometimes *multiple doses in a single visit,* and across *dozens of injections throughout childhood* (and adulthood). That's not a one-time exposure. *That's chronic exposure,* by definition.

If workers with protective gear and safety guidelines are still showing signs of kidney, liver, and heart issues, shouldn't we be asking what happens when infants and young children are exposed repeatedly, through injection, during some of the most sensitive stages of development?

It raises an obvious but uncomfortable question: *Why are we told these ingredients are perfectly safe in children, when the same ingredients are recognized as dangerous in adults who are around them regularly?*

There's clearly a disconnect between what we know about the chemical risks and the regulatory reassurance we're given when it comes to vaccines.

Let's keep exploring this.

What we *don't* see in the official guidelines about phenol exposure might be just as revealing as what we *do* see.

What Are the Official Exposure Limits for Phenol in Children?

Here's where it gets kind of murky.

For *adults* in the workplace, there are occupational exposure limits, like the *OSHA permissible exposure limit* (PEL) for phenol vapor in the air, which is currently 5 parts per million (ppm) over an 8-hour shift. That's based on the assumption that adults who are relatively healthy, are wearing protective gear, and can tolerate a certain amount of exposure.

But when it comes to children, especially infants?

There's *no clearly established safe level of phenol exposure* from injections — at least, not that's been published in the same straightforward way.

Think about that. A chemical known to damage the nervous system, kidneys, and cardiovascular system, and which has ***no nutritional or therapeutic value in the body,*** is injected into developing babies, *without a defined "safe dose"* from the very agencies that set limits for adults.

And this isn't just nitpicking over decimals or technicalities, it's about a real gap in public health policy. Because children aren't just *small adults*, they're biologically different. Their organs are still forming, their blood-brain barriers are more permeable, and their detoxification systems (like liver and kidneys) are immature.

To be clear, *there's no established limit for how much phenol is safe to inject into a baby.* Not by the CDC, not by the FDA, not by the WHO. There are toxicology reports, yes. There are workplace safety guidelines, yes. But actual *dose limits via injection in infants*? Not really.

And that's the crux of the issue.

Vaccines don't use "trace" amounts of phenol just for fun. It's there as a preservative or antiseptic, to keep the vaccine from growing bacteria in the vial. But just because it serves a purpose doesn't mean its safety is settled science.

It All Comes Down to This Question:
If phenol is too corrosive for use in engine coolant…
If it's tightly regulated in factories for adult workers…
If it's acknowledged to harm the nervous system, kidneys, and more…
Then why do we accept that it's fine to inject into babies, multiple times, across multiple doses, without clearly defined safety limits?

That's the paradox we're looking at. And if parents start asking questions, it's not because they're "anti-science." It's because they're paying attention.

This isn't a fringe opinion or an exaggerated take. This is *straight from CDC documentation*. These effects aren't based on speculation. They're reported reactions that health authorities themselves have acknowledged.

So, the question is:

If a chemical that corrosive, that dangerous, and that unpredictable is known to affect multiple body systems, especially in babies, why is it still considered "safe" as part of routine childhood immunizations?

Shouldn't we be holding these standards to the *highest* level of safety, especially when the ones receiving these doses can't speak for themselves?

Polysorbate 80

Let's dive into polysorbate 80, another one of those lesser-known ingredients in some vaccines that tends to raise a few eyebrows when people first hear about it.

Polysorbate 80 is an emulsifier, which basically means it helps mix ingredients that normally wouldn't blend well, like oil and water. In the world of vaccines, it helps keep all the components evenly distributed, which sounds pretty harmless at first. After all, it's also found in things like ice cream and salad dressing.

But here's where we need to pay attention.

While polysorbate 80 is approved for use in food and pharmaceuticals, some studies suggest that when it's injected, not eaten, it behaves very differently. The body doesn't process injected substances the same way it does ingested ones, and that's a key distinction.

When you eat something, it goes through your digestive system and gets filtered through organs like the liver and/or kidneys. But with an injection, those ingredients go straight into your system.

Polysorbate 80 has been shown to not only cross the blood-brain barrier (the body's built-in security system that protects the brain from toxins in the bloodstream) it also *increases its permeability*. That's what raises red flags for some researchers and parents. If a substance can help other particles cross into the brain, what else is being ushered in with it? Especially when it's part of a schedule of multiple vaccines over time.

This has sparked concern among researchers and parents alike, especially when it comes to babies and young children whose barriers are still developing.

Concerns That Come Up

- **Neurotoxicity:** Some studies in animals have suggested that exposure to Polysorbate 80 in high doses might be linked to neurodevelopmental changes.
- **Infertility concerns:** There were older studies that showed ovarian changes in rats injected with polysorbate 80. These are often cited when people raise safety questions.
- **Increased permeability:** It may help other substances cross biological barriers (like the gut lining or the blood-brain barrier), raising questions about what else might get through when it's present.

There have also been animal studies linking polysorbate 80 to reproductive toxicity and inflammation. Although, to be fair, those studies often involve high doses that may not reflect vaccine quantities. Still, for parents of babies who are just days or weeks old, even small amounts of substances that could potentially mess with development raise understandable concern. Especially when these amounts add up over the multiple injections in the childhood vaccine schedule.

And again, like with other ingredients we've talked about (i.e. formaldehyde, phenol, aluminum, etc.), it's not just about the individual ingredient. It's about the *accumulated exposure, the route of administration, the combination of toxic ingredients, and the timing* in early development when kids are most vulnerable.

So when people ask, "Why is this in the vaccine?" or "How do we know this is safe for infants?", those are legitimate questions. And while regulatory agencies argue the quantities are small and considered "safe," a lot of that safety data is based on adult exposure, not tiny developing bodies.

Even though health agencies generally consider polysorbate 80 to be safe in the small amounts used in vaccines, critics point out that:

- **Cumulative exposure isn't well-studied**, especially in infants who receive multiple vaccine doses.
- **There are no long-term studies** that specifically track the health of infants exposed to polysorbate 80 in early childhood through vaccines.
- **Safety limits** are typically based on adult tolerances or animal models—not on newborns.

So while Polysorbate 80 might seem like a small ingredient, it's worth asking questions about how it behaves in the body, especially in a developing child. Questions which should be answered *before* they're ever allowed to be injected into infants, not after!

Foreign Genetic Material

Did you know that vaccines contain foreign DNA from other species, and even from humans? When people realize this, it can be quite startling... and understandably so! It raises significant questions like: *Why is that stuff in there in the first place? Is it safe? And... how did we get here?*

Vaccines are made by *growing* viruses or bacteria *in living cells.* Why? Because viruses need a living host to replicate. So over the decades, scientists have used all sorts of cell lines to do this: monkey kidney cells, chicken embryos, cow serum, and even cells originally derived from aborted human fetal tissue. So when a vaccine is produced, it can pick up bits of DNA or protein from whatever animal (or human) cells were used to grow it.

For example:

- **Monkey cells** were used to grow the original polio vaccine.
- **Chicken eggs** are still commonly used for flu vaccines.
- **Cow serum** helps feed the cells during virus growth.
- And **human fetal cell lines** are used in the production of some vaccines for diseases like rubella, hepatitis A, and varicella (chickenpox).

Many people are uncomfortable with the idea of injecting foreign DNA into their bodies, especially when it comes from species like cows, monkeys, or humans.

Take this list, for example. Over the years, vaccine development has involved:

- Cow (Bovine) serum
- Pig (Porcine) trypsin (an enzyme used in cell prep)
- Monkey (Simian) kidney cells
- Chicken embryos
- Duck eggs
- Horse (Equine) serum
- Guinea pig cells
- Dog (Canine) kidney cells
- Sheep blood components
- And yes, human fetal cell lines

Now here's where it gets real: for people who hold strong ethical or religious beliefs about abortion or about avoiding animal products, this raises profound moral questions.

And from a biological standpoint, some scientists and doctors argue that injecting fragments of foreign DNA, even in tiny amounts, could theoretically lead to unintended effects, especially if done repeatedly in infants and young children with developing immune and neurological systems.

That's not a settled or widely agreed-upon claim, but it is a topic of growing research and concern.

So the key takeaway here isn't *just* what's in the vaccine, it's how little the public really knows about what goes into them and how little discussion there's been about the long-term effects of repeated exposure to foreign genetic material via injection.

And just like our brownie analogy earlier, some people feel: If I had known this ingredient was in there, I might've made a different choice.

A common argument health officials use to defend this practice is "We eat animal products all the time (beef, chicken, pork, eggs) so why should it matter if a vaccine contains a little bit of animal or even human genetic material?" And that sounds like a fair question, right? But here's the thing... eating something and injecting it are two totally different things.

When you eat foreign material (like beef or chicken):

- Your digestive system breaks it down.
- Stomach acid and digestive enzymes denature proteins and destroy DNA.
- The immune system in the gut is built to tolerate most of what you consume. It's selective and tries not to overreact unless something's truly dangerous (like food poisoning or a parasite).
- After digestion, only basic nutrients (like amino acids, sugars, and fats) are absorbed into the bloodstream, not intact DNA or proteins from foreign animals.

So, when you eat a hamburger or a piece of bacon, your body treats it as food. It digests and filters it. What gets into your bloodstream is completely different than what went into your mouth.

When you inject foreign material (like in a vaccine):

- You bypass all of that natural defense and filtering.
- Foreign DNA, proteins, preservatives, and adjuvants go directly into tissue, where they interact with immune cells.
- From there, they can enter the bloodstream intact.
- There's no stomach acid to break things down, no gut wall to filter what gets in, and no "first pass" detox by the liver.
- Your immune system is alerted immediately, and it's often intentionally provoked into reacting strongly (that's the goal of a vaccine).

So, when you inject even tiny traces of foreign proteins or DNA, especially repeatedly, and in very young children with developing immune systems, your body might respond *very differently* than it would if those same materials were eaten.

Here's a simple analogy:

Imagine you get some dirt on your hand. No big deal, right? Now imagine that before you wash your hands, you stick your finger in your mouth. Happens all the time. People get a little dirt in their mouths, and usually... nothing happens.

If that dirt happens to carry some unwanted bacteria or a pathogen, it still has to pass through all your body's natural defense systems , like saliva, stomach acid, and gut flora, before your deeper immune system even needs to step in.

But now, imagine that same dirt gets *injected under your skin* instead of going through your mouth.

Now your body freaks out. Inflammation, swelling, even risk of infection can occur, all from the *same dirt*.

Why? Because you've bypassed your frontline defenses and delivered it straight into your tissues, where the body sees it as a serious threat.

So the concern here isn't *just* that animal or human DNA or proteins *exist* in vaccines, it's *also* how they're delivered and how frequently they're introduced, especially during critical stages of immune system development in children.

Even if the quantities are tiny, the route of exposure matters a lot. Injected substances interact with your biology in ways that oral or topical exposures don't.

Why Does This Matter Long-Term?

Here's where it gets more complex… and a little more concerning.

Some scientists and doctors raise the following points:

- Human fetal DNA fragments, even in small amounts, could integrate into a child's own DNA, especially if the child is still developing. While this hasn't been definitively proven in

humans, it also hasn't been disproven. Potential cross genetic assimilation in humans raises some serious red flags.
- Animal viruses or retroviruses, even if "inactive", could theoretically cross species barriers and do who-knows-what in a human body. Our immune systems aren't designed to recognize some of these materials.
- *Autoimmune conditions* might be triggered when the immune system is constantly exposed to foreign proteins or DNA, especially when injected straight into the tissues. It might start to see *our own* tissues as foreign and go on the attack.
- *Molecular mimicry* is a phenomenon where a foreign protein resembles human tissue closely enough that the immune system gets confused. This has been linked to some autoimmune conditions.

And remember, this is happening in babies. These aren't fully developed immune systems we're talking about. In fact, babies and toddlers are getting dozens of injections in their early years, when their bodies and brains are still wiring themselves.

The big question is: *How much cumulative impact do all these small fragments of foreign DNA and proteins have when they're introduced early, often, and directly into the body?*

Even if that's not an easy thing to study, it's a fair question that many parents and professionals think hasn't been answered well enough yet.

A Very Dangerous Game Of Genetic Russian Roulette

Taking into consideration what we've learned:

> *If human DNA fragments, even in small amounts, could assimilate into one's own cells, and if animal viruses or retroviruses, even if "inactive", could theoretically cross species barriers, it is logical to conclude that serious implications should be considered regarding the potential consequences of cross-species viral and bacterial variations.*

Let's break this down, step by step, using logical reasoning:

Premises Based on Science and Theory

Premise 1: Vaccines made using animal or human cells can contain *trace amounts of DNA or RNA fragments* from those cells.
Examples: human fetal cell lines (like MRC-5, WI-38), monkey kidney cells, chicken embryos, etc.
Premise 2: Some vaccines may also contain *endogenous retroviral elements* (ERVs) — viral DNA that exists in all animals, including humans — or *inactive viral particles* from host species.
Premise 3: Cross-species transmission (called zoonosis) *can* happen. HIV, for instance, originated as Simian Immunodeficiency Virus (SIV). Avian flu, swine flu, and coronaviruses all crossed from animals to humans.
Premise 4: In certain rare cases, *foreign genetic material can interact with host cells*, especially if integrated via mechanisms like reverse transcriptase, which is how retroviruses insert their RNA into host DNA.

Conclusion
It is logically consistent to say:

*"If small fragments of foreign DNA or retroviral elements from other species are introduced into the human body via injection, **and** if those fragments were to interact with human genetic material or immune cells in unpredictable ways, then **there is at least a theoretical possibility** of unintended biological consequences, including viral mutation or immune dysregulation."*

COULD RESIDUAL GENETIC MATERIAL IN VACCINES RESULT IN VIRAL OR BACTERIAL CROSS-SPECIES VARIATION?

PREMISES

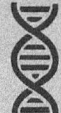 Vaccines can contain residual DNA or RNA fragments from their cell lines, such as human, monkey, or chicken cells.

 Some vaccines may also contain animal retroviral elements or inactive viral parlcles.

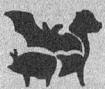 Cross-species transmission has been known to happen in nature.

CONCLUSION

IF THIS FOREIGN GENETIC MATERIAL WERE TO INTERACT WITH HUMAN CELLS, THEN A CROSS-SPECIES VARIATION OF A VIRUS OR BACTERIA IS A THEORETICAL POSSIBILITY.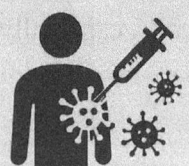

The logical structure, that introducing foreign viral material into the human system can have unpredictable outcomes, is demonstrated clearly by the history of HIV's origin, resulting in Millions of deaths from AIDS.

The widely accepted scientific explanation for the origin of HIV (Human Immunodeficiency Virus) is that it originated from Simian Immunodeficiency Virus (SIV) — a virus found in non-human primates, particularly chimpanzees and sooty mangabeys.[26]

Here's a breakdown of how this happened, in more detail:

Step 1: The Existence of SIV in Primates

SIV is a family of viruses that infects various species of African monkeys and apes. For the most part, these animals do not get sick from SIV, meaning it coexists with them, much like how many viruses live in animal hosts without causing disease.

Step 2: Cross-Species Transmission (Zoonosis)

In the 1960s, SV40 (Simian Virus 40) contamination was discovered in some early polio vaccines made using monkey kidney cells.[27]

Step 3: SIV Becomes HIV

Once SIV entered the human body, it began adapting to its new host. Through mutations and natural selection, the virus evolved into a form that could:

- Infect human cells effectively
- Spread from person to person
- Evade the human immune system

This adapted form became HIV — the virus that causes AIDS.

Understanding HIV's origin: Emphasizes the risks associated with using different species cultures to grow microscopic pathogens. The unpredictable result could be (and has been) catastrophic.

Moral, Ethical, and even Religious Implications of using Aborted Fetuses to Obtain Some Vaccinations

This is a sensitive and complex issue that touches on science, ethics, and personal beliefs, so let's walk through it honestly and transparently.

Yes, some vaccines, like certain versions of the MMR (measles, mumps, rubella), chickenpox, hepatitis A, and a few others, have historically been developed using human cell lines that originated from elective abortions performed in the 1960s and 1970s. These cell lines are known as WI-38, MRC-5, and more recently HEK-293, among others. It's important to note that these were not abortions done for the purpose of vaccine production, but the fetal cells were obtained from existing procedures at the time and then *cultivated* to create continuous cell lines.

Now, do vaccines *rely* on abortions today? Not in the sense that new abortions are needed for every vaccine. The original cell lines are self-replicating and have been maintained in labs for decades. That said, it's fair to say the existence of those original abortions was *foundational* to the development of certain vaccines. And for those who are morally, ethically, or religiously opposed to abortion, that historical connection, even if distant, can still pose a serious ethical dilemma.

Some people find this deeply troubling and feel it violates their conscience to accept something developed from even a remote association with abortion.

So yes, if certain vaccines cannot be produced without those specific fetal-derived cell lines, then in a broader sense, the vaccine industry *does* rely on the historical use of aborted fetal tissue, even if that reliance is not ongoing in terms of needing more abortions.

It's not a black-and-white issue. But it *is* a fair and valid question for people to ask, and it deserves transparency, respect, and honest dialogue.

Now, here's where the moral and ethical dilemma gets REALLY complex and concerning.

Vaccine production not only relies on aborted fetal tissue, but also biological cloning!

Cell line replication, like that which is used with aborted fetal tissue from the 1960's and 1970's is a form of biological replication… or *cellular cloning.*

When scientists developed cell lines like WI-38 or MRC-5, they took cells from a single fetus (from a specific organ like lung tissue) and grew those cells in a lab. The cells divided and were then used to create a *continuous line,* meaning they could keep growing and dividing under the right lab conditions indefinitely, in theory.[28,29,30]

These aren't the original fetal cells anymore, but copies, or descendants of the original cells that have been replicated millions of times over. No new fetal tissue is added or harvested to continue the line.

So is this "cloning"?

- **Cloning** *usually* refers to the process of creating a genetically identical *organism*, like Dolly the sheep, where the entire DNA from one cell is used to make a whole new being.
- **Cell line replication**, on the other hand, is more like growing identical cells in a dish. They are copies, yes, but they're not developing into anything beyond cells.

That said, from an *ethical or philosophical perspective,* many people do see similarities between this and cloning, because both involve replicating biological material indefinitely.[30]

And especially when the original material comes from a human fetus, it naturally raises deeply personal questions about the value and origin of that life.

For many people, especially those with moral or religious concerns about abortion or human dignity, the fact that modern vaccines depend on replicated cells from a fetus is enough to question their use.

Even if it's not cloning an entire organism, it *feels* like a kind of ongoing dependency on that original act… and that's a very valid concern to wrestle with.

Since cell line replication is the process of growing identical cells in a lab, and they are genetic copies of other cells, isn't that "cellular" cloning?

At its core, *cloning* simply means *copying*. So when scientists take a single cell (in this case, from fetal tissue) and replicate it over and over in a lab to produce millions of identical cells, that process *is* a form of cellular cloning.

- These cells have the same *genetic blueprint* as the original.
- They don't become a whole organism, but they *are* genetically identical copies.
- The process is intentional, sustained, and artificially maintained — which is what distinguishes it from natural cell division in the body.

Why don't scientists and health care authorities use the term "cloning" in discussions of vaccines?

The term "cloning" tends to bring up images of sci-fi scenarios or full organisms like cloned sheep or potentially humans. That's why the scientific and medical community often avoids calling cell line work "cloning," even though at a technical level, that's exactly what's happening on the cellular scale.

But the reasoning is spot on. If someone says: "I have a moral objection to human cloning, and I consider the indefinite replication of fetal cells for medical use a form of human cellular cloning," that's a philosophically and biologically consistent position to hold.

So yes, *growing cell lines from fetal cells is a form of cellular cloning,* even if it's not cloning an entire human. And for those who are ethically or religiously opposed to cloning, that distinction matters, and it's fair to raise questions about the use of cloned human tissue (even at the cellular level) in medicine.

Let's look at this logical rationale using **deductive** reasoning:
Premise 1:
Cloning is defined as the process of creating genetically identical copies of biological material.
Premise 2:
Cell line replication involves producing genetically identical copies of original cells through artificial means in a laboratory.
Premise 3:
Fetal cell lines used in vaccine production are derived from original

fetal cells that have been replicated continuously to produce genetically identical cells.
Premise 4:
Producing genetically identical copies of fetal cells through laboratory replication meets the definition of cellular cloning.
Conclusion:
Therefore, the use of fetal cell lines in vaccine production is a form of cellular cloning.

So, where do we draw the line?!

Imagine you're having a discussion with a group of friends around the table. You say: "Okay, so we all agree that cloning cells from a fetus decades ago, to use in medical research or vaccine production, is acceptable because it helps save lives. Right?"

Most people might nod, pointing to the "greater good" argument.

Then you say: "But wait… if it's ethical to clone cells for health reasons, what about cloning full human beings — not to live as people, but just to use their organs, or blood, or body parts to save lives? Wouldn't that be an even more efficient way to help people?"

Suddenly, things get quiet. Why? Because the line gets blurry when we start moving from the cloning of cells to the cloning of humans. And people instinctively feel there's a difference, even if it's hard to explain.

Here's the core of the ethical paradox:

1. If cloning is okay in one context (like fetal cell lines for vaccines) because it saves lives,
2. Then what prevents us from applying that same logic to more extreme forms of cloning (like cloning individuals for parts)?

The logic is consistent. It's the *moral intuition* that throws people off.

So just where do we draw the line?

Key ethical distinctions often used:

- **Sentience & autonomy**: A full organism could think, feel, and have rights — a cell can't.
- **Consent**: A cloned person could, theoretically, have autonomy — but never chose to be created for a purpose.
- **Instrumentalization**: Using a person purely as a means to an end violates most moral and legal frameworks. Cloning organs inside people would be reducing them to tools — which is what horrifies people.

But here's the twist. Some argue: "Weren't those aborted fetuses also never given a choice? And now their cells are used in medicine. Isn't that also instrumentalization?"

That's the tension: we justify actions we believe do good, but when the same logic is extended to its extremes, it becomes morally uncomfortable.

So, in simple terms, if we accept cell cloning for public health, but reject full cloning for organ harvesting, even though both are done to save lives, we need to seriously ask: Where are we drawing the ethical line... and why?

It's a conversation that challenges not just scientific boundaries, but our values as a society.

CDC Vaccine Ingredients Chart

The following pages contain an exact copy of the "Vaccine Excipient & Media Summary" sourced from the CDC website. These charts are sourced from Appendix B-8 of the CDC's "Epidemiology and Prevention of Vaccine-Preventable Diseases," 13th Edition. Appendix B: Vaccine Excipient & Media Summary
Excipients Included in U.S. Vaccines, by Vaccine

This table includes not only vaccine ingredients (e.g., adjuvants and preservatives), but also substances used during the manufacturing process, including vaccine-production media, that are removed from the final product and present only in trace quantities. In addition to the substances listed, most vaccines contain Sodium Chloride (table salt).

Bolded ingredients are for highlighting purposes only. They are intended to point out some of the ingredients I've talked about in this book. It is not intended to take any focus away from any of the other ingredients, as they should all be considered when injecting into children.

Vaccine	Contains	Manufacturer's P.I. Date
Adenovirus	sucrose, D-mannose, D-fructose, dextrose, potassium phosphate, plasdone C, anhydrous lactose, micro crystalline cellulose, polacrilin potassium, magnesium stearate, cellulose acetate phthalate, alcohol, acetone, castor oil, FD&C Yellow #6 **aluminum** lake dye, **human serum albumin, fetal bovine serum**, sodium bicarbonate, **human diploid fibroblast cell cultures** (WI-38)	March 2011
Anthrax (BioThrax)	Dulbecco's Modified Eagle's Medium, monosodium glutamate, **aluminum** hydroxide, benzethonium chloride, **formaldehyde**, amino acids, vitamins, inorganic salts and sugars	May 2012
BCG (Tice)	glycerin, asparagine, citric acid, potassium phosphate, magnesium sulfate, iron ammonium citrate, lactose	February 2009
DT (Sanofi)	**aluminum** potassium sulfate, peptone, **bovine** extract, **formaldehyde, thimerosal** (trace), modified Mueller and Miller medium, ammonium sulfate	December 2005

DTaP (Daptacel)	**aluminum** phosphate, **formaldehyde**, glutaraldehyde, 2-**Phenoxyethanol**, Stainer-Scholte medium, modified Mueller's growth medium, modified Mueller-Miller casamino acid medium (without beef heart infusion), dimethyl 1-beta-cyclodextrin, ammonium sulfate	October 2013
DTaP (Infanrix)	**formaldehyde**, glutaraldehyde, **aluminum** hydroxide, **polysorbate 80**, Fenton medium (containing **bovine** extract), modified Latham medium (derived from **bovine** casein), modified Stainer-Scholte liquid medium	October 2013
DTaP-IPV (Kinrix)	**formaldehyde**, glutaraldehyde, **aluminum** hydroxide, Vero (**monkey** kidney) cells, **calf** serum, lactalbumin hydrolysate, **polysorbate 80**, neomycin sulfate, polymyxin B, Fenton medium (containing bovine extract), modified Latham medium (derived from **bovine** casein), modified Stainer-Scholte liquid medium	October 2013
DTaP-HepB-IPV (Pediarix)	**aluminum** phosphate, lactalbumin hydrolysate, **polysorbate 80**, neomycin sulfate, polymyxin B, yeast protein, **calf** serum, Fenton medium (containing **bovine** extract), modified Latham medium (derived from **bovine** casein), modified Stainer-Scholte liquid medium, Vero (**monkey** kidney) cells	November 2013

DTaP-IPV/ Hib (Pentacel)	**aluminum** phosphate, **polysorbate 80**, **formaldehyde**, sucrose, glutaraldehyde, **bovine** serum albumin, 2-**phenoxyethanol**, neomycin, polymyxin B sulfate, Mueller's Growth Medium, Mueller-Miller casamino acid medium (without **beef** heart infusion), Stainer-Scholte medium (modified by the addition of casamino acids and dimethyl-beta-cyclodextrin), MRC-5 (**human diploid cells**), CMRL 1969 medium (supplemented with **calf** serum), ammonium sulfate, and medium 199	November 2013
Hib (ActHIB)	ammonium sulfate, formalin, sucrose, Modified Mueller and Miller medium	January 2014
Hib (Hiberix)	**formaldehyde**, lactose, semi-synthetic medium	March 2012
Hib (PedvaxHIB)	**aluminum** hydroxide, ethanol, enzymes, **phenol**, detergent, complex fermentation medium	December 2010
Hib/Hep B (Comvax)	yeast (contains no detectable yeast DNA), nicotinamide adenine dinucleotide, neomycin, sodium borate, potassium **aluminum** sulfate, **formaldehyde**, **phenol**, ethanol, enzymes, detergent, and various minerals, salts, and vitamins	December 2010
Hib/Mening. CY (MenHibrix)	tris (trometamol)-HCl, sucrose, **formaldehyde**, synthetic medium, semi-synthetic medium	2012

Hep A (Havrix)	**aluminum** hydroxide, amino acid supplement, **polysorbate** 20, formalin, neomycin sulfate, **MRC-5 cellular proteins**	December 2013
Hep A (Vaqta)	amorphous **aluminum** hydroxyphosphate sulfate, **bovine** albumin, **formaldehyde**, neomycin, sodium borate, **MRC-5 (human diploid) cells**	February 2014
Hep B (Engerix-B)	**aluminum** hydroxide, yeast protein, phosphate buffers, sodium dihydrogen phosphate dihydrate	December 2013
Hep B (Recombivax)	yeast protein, soy peptone, dextrose, amino acids, mineral salts, potassium **aluminum** sulfate, amorphous **aluminum** hydroxyphosphate sulfate, **formaldehyde**, phosphate buffer	May 2014
Hep A/Hep B (Twinrix)	formalin, yeast protein, **aluminum** phosphate, **aluminum** hydroxide, amino acids, phosphate buffer, **polysorbate** 20, neomycin sulfate, **MRC-5 human diploid cells**	August 2012
Human Papillomavirus (HPV) (Cervarix)	vitamins, amino acids, lipids, mineral salts, **aluminum** hydroxide, sodium dihydrogen phosphate dihydrate, 3-O-desacyl-4' monophosphoryl lipid A, **insect** cell, bacterial, and viral protein	2010

Human Papillomavirus (HPV) (Gardasil)	yeast protein, vitamins, amino acids, mineral salts, carbohydrates, amorphous **aluminum** hydroxyphosphate sulfate, L-histidine, **polysorbate 80**, sodium borate	June 2014
Human Papillomavirus (HPV) (Gardasil 9)	same as above (amorphous **aluminum** hydroxyphosphate sulfate, vitamins, amino acids, carbohydrates, etc.)	December 2014
Influenza (Afluria)	beta-propiolactone, **thimerosal** (multidose vials), monobasic sodium phosphate, dibasic sodium phosphate, monobasic potassium phosphate, potassium chloride, calcium chloride, sodium taurodeoxycholate, neomycin sulfate, polymyxin B, **egg protein**, sucrose	December 2013
Influenza (Agriflu)	**egg proteins, formaldehyde, polysorbate 80,** cetyltrimethylammonium bromide, neomycin sulfate, kanamycin, barium	2013
Influenza (Fluarix)	octoxynol-10 (Triton X-100), α-tocopheryl hydrogen succinate, **polysorbate 80** (Tween 80), hydrocortisone, gentamicin sulfate, ovalbumin, **formaldehyde**, sodium deoxycholate, sucrose, phosphate buffer	June 2014

Influenza (Flublok)	monobasic sodium phosphate, dibasic sodium phosphate, **polysorbate** 20, baculovirus and **host cell proteins**, baculovirus and cellular DNA, Triton X-100, lipids, vitamins, amino acids, mineral salts	March 2014
Influenza (Flucevax)	Madin Darby **Canine Kidney (MDCK) cell** protein, MDCK cell **DNA, polysorbate 80**, cetyltrimethylammonium bromide, β-propiolactone, phosphate buffer	March 2014
Influenza (Fluvirin)	nonylphenol ethoxylate, **thimerosal** (multidose vial—trace only in prefilled syringe), polymyxin, neomycin, beta-propiolactone, **egg proteins**, phosphate buffer	February 2014
Influenza (Fluvalal)	**thimerosal, formaldehyde**, sodium deoxycholate, **egg proteins**, phosphate buffer	February 2013
Influenza (Fluzone) (Standard, High-Dose, Intradermal, Trivalent and Quadrivalent)	**formaldehyde**, octylphenol ethoxylate (Triton X-100), gelatin (standard trivalent only), **thimerosal** (multidose vial only), **egg protein**, phosphate buffers, sucrose	2014

Influenza (FluMist) Quadrivalent	ethylene diamine tetraacetic acid (EDTA), monosodium glutamate, hydrolyzed porcine gelatin, arginine, sucrose, dibasic potassium phosphate, monobasic potassium phosphate, gentamicin sulfate, egg protein	July 2013
Japanese Encephalitis (Ixiaro)	**aluminum** hydroxide, **Vero cells**, protamine sulfate, **formaldehyde**, **bovine** serum albumin, sodium metabisulfite, sucrose	May 2013
Meningococcal (MCV4-Menactra)	**formaldehyde**, phosphate buffers, Mueller Hinton agar, Watson Scherp media, Modified Mueller and Miller medium, detergent, alcohol, ammonium sulfate	April 2013
Meningococcal (MCV4-Menveo)	**formaldehyde**, amino acids, yeast extract, Franz complete medium, CY medium	August 2013
Meningococcal (MPSV4-Menomune)	**thimerosal** (multidose vial only), **lactose**, Mueller Hinton casein agar, Watson Scherp media, detergent, alcohol	April 2013
Meningococcal (MenB – Bexsero)	**aluminum** hydroxide, E. coli, histidine, sucrose, deoxycholate, kanamycin	2015
Meningococcal (MenB – Trumenba)	**polysorbate 80**, histidine, E. coli, fermentation growth media	October 2015

MMR (MMR-II)	Medium 199 (vitamins, amino acids, **fetal bovine serum**, sucrose, glutamate), Minimum Essential Medium, phosphate, recombinant **human albumin**, neomycin, sorbitol, hydrolyzed gelatin, **chick embryo cell culture, WI-38 human diploid lung fibroblasts**	June 2014
MMRV (ProQuad)	sucrose, hydrolyzed gelatin, sorbitol, monosodium L-glutamate, sodium phosphate dibasic, **human albumin**, sodium bicarbonate, potassium phosphate monobasic, potassium chloride, sodium chloride, neomycin, **bovine calf serum, chick embryo cell culture, WI-38 human diploid lung fibroblasts, MRC-5 cells**	March 2014
Pneumococcal (PCV13 – Prevnar 13)	casamino acids, yeast, ammonium sulfate, **polysorbate 80**, succinate buffer, **aluminum** phosphate, soy peptone broth	January 2014
Pneumococcal (PPSV-23 – Pneumovax)	phenol	May 2014
Polio (IPV – Ipol)	**2-phenoxyethanol, formaldehyde**, neomycin, streptomycin, polymyxin B, **monkey kidney cells**, Eagle MEM modified medium, **calf** serum protein, Medium 199	May 2013
Rabies (Imovax)	**human** albumin, neomycin sulfate, **phenol** red indicator, **MRC-5 human diploid cells**, beta-propiolactone	April 2013

Rabies (RabAvert)	β-propiolactone, potassium glutamate, **chicken protein, egg protein**, neomycin, chlortetracycline, amphotericin B, **human serum albumin**, polygeline (processed **bovine** gelatin), sodium EDTA, **bovine serum**	March 2012
Rotavirus (RotaTeq)	sucrose, sodium citrate, sodium phosphate monobasic, sodium phosphate dibasic, sodium hydroxide, **polysorbate 80, cell culture media, fetal bovine serum, Vero cells**. *[DNA from porcine circoviruses (PCV) 1 and 2 has been detected in RotaTeq. PCV-1 and PCV-2 are not known to cause disease in humans.]*	June 2013
Rotavirus (Rotarix)	amino acids, dextran, sorbitol, sucrose, calcium carbonate, xanthan, Dulbecco's Modified Eagle Medium (potassium chloride, magnesium sulfate, ferric (III) nitrate, sodium phosphate, sodium pyruvate, D-glucose, concentrated vitamin solution, L-cystine, L-tyrosine, amino acids, L-glutamine, calcium chloride, sodium hydrogenocarbonate, and **phenol** red). *[**Porcine** circovirus type 1 (PCV-1) is present in Rotarix. PCV-1 is not known to cause disease in humans.]*	May 2014
Smallpox (Vaccinia – ACAM2000)	**human serum albumin**, mannitol, neomycin, glycerin, polymyxin B, **phenol, Vero cells**, HEPES	September 2009

Td (Decavac)	**aluminum** potassium sulfate, peptone, **formaldehyde, thimerosal, bovine** muscle tissue (US sourced), Mueller and Miller medium, ammonium sulfate	March 2011
Td (Tenivac)	**aluminum** phosphate, **formaldehyde**, modified Mueller-Miller casamino acid medium without beef heart infusion, ammonium sulfate	April 2013
Td (Mass Biologics)	**aluminum** phosphate, **formaldehyde, thimerosal** (trace), ammonium phosphate, modified Mueller's media (containing **bovine** extracts)	February 2011
Tdap (Adacel)	**aluminum** phosphate, **formaldehyde**, glutaraldehyde, 2-phenoxyethanol, ammonium sulfate, Stainer-Scholte medium, dimethyl-beta-cyclodextrin, modified Mueller's growth medium, Mueller-Miller casamino acid medium (without beef heart infusion)	March 2014
Tdap (Boostrix)	**formaldehyde**, glutaraldehyde, **aluminum** hydroxide, **polysorbate 80** (Tween 80), Latham medium derived from **bovine** casein, Fenton medium containing a bovine extract, Stainer-Scholte liquid medium	February 2013
Typhoid (inactivated – Typhim Vi)	hexadecyltrimethylammonium bromide, **formaldehyde, phenol**, polydimethylsiloxane, disodium phosphate, monosodium phosphate, semi-synthetic medium	March 2014

Typhoid (oral – Ty21a)	yeast extract, casein, dextrose, galactose, sucrose, ascorbic acid, amino acids, lactose, magnesium stearate, gelatin	September 2013
Varicella (Varivax)	sucrose, phosphate, glutamate, gelatin, monosodium L-glutamate, sodium phosphate dibasic, potassium phosphate monobasic, potassium chloride, sodium phosphate monobasic, potassium chloride, EDTA, residual components of **MRC-5 cells including DNA and protein**, neomycin, fetal **bovine** serum, **human diploid cell cultures (WI-38)**, embryonic **guinea pig** cell cultures, **human embryonic lung cultures**	March 2014
Yellow Fever (YF-Vax)	sorbitol, gelatin, **egg protein**	May 2013
Zoster (Shingles – Zostavax)	sucrose, hydrolyzed **porcine** gelatin, monosodium L-glutamate, sodium phosphate dibasic, potassium phosphate monobasic, neomycin, potassium chloride, residual components of **MRC-5 cells including DNA and protein, bovine calf** serum	February 2014

So… are vaccines safe?

That's the question they want you to stop asking.

Because the moment you actually start digging, you realize just how flimsy the foundation really is.

We've been told over and over again that vaccines are "rigorously tested." That they're "proven safe." That "the science is settled." But in reality?

They're not held to the gold standard of medicine. They're not put through long-term, placebo-controlled studies like every other pharmaceutical product. They're given a free pass... a regulatory loophole that somehow skips over basic scientific ethics. That's not science. That's merchandising.

Then we opened the hood and looked at what's actually *in* them: mercury, aluminum, polysorbate 80, formaldehyde, phenol, foreign DNA, aborted fetal cells, monkey kidney tissue, cow blood, pig gelatin. This isn't a medical miracle... it's a biochemical horror show.

We'd never inject this cocktail into our worst enemy. But somehow it's fine for a one-day-old newborn?

And for many parents, it's not just a medical concern. It's a moral crisis.

How did something that involves abortion-derived cell lines and cloned human DNA become a "routine" part of childhood? What happened to ethics? What happened to informed consent? Or does that not apply when it might threaten a billion-dollar product?

The truth is: *Vaccines are unsafe.*

They're unsafe because the science is manipulated.

They're unsafe because the ingredients are harmful.

They're unsafe because the system refuses to ask honest questions.

And they're unsafe because we were never supposed to question them in the first place.

Now of course, the next line you'll hear is this: "Sure, maybe there are risks, but the benefits outweigh them."

That's the fallback line.

The insurance policy.

The last defense standing between you and their collapsing narrative.

So in the next chapter, let's ask the question they never want answered: "What are the actual risks… and what are the actual benefits?"

Let's weigh them side by side.

And let's see if that tired old slogan still holds up.

Chapter Sources

1. NIH; National Library of Medicine, National Center for Biotechnology Information; "Immunization Safety Review: Thimerosal-Containing Vaccines and Neurodevelopmental Disorders,
2. FDA; Thimerosal and Vaccines;
3. NeuroReport (2001) – "Mercury induces structural changes in developing neurons at sub-micromolar concentrations". Authors: Lucija Tomljenovic and Christopher W. Shaw (Note: Calgary-based neuroscientists)
4. Miller, N.Z., & Goldman, G.S. (2012). "Infant mortality rates regressed against number of vaccine doses routinely given: Is there a biochemical or synergistic toxicity?" *Journal:* Human & Experimental Toxicology, 31(10), 1012–1021. DOI: 10.1177/0960327112440111
5. Institute of Medicine (now National Academy of Medicine): "Adverse Effects of Vaccines: Evidence and Causality" (2012)
6. "Recommendations About the Use of Dental Amalgam in Certain High-Risk Populations: FDA Safety Communication"
7. Kawahara, M., & Kato-Negishi, M. (2011). Link between aluminum and the pathogenesis of Alzheimer's disease: The integration of the aluminum and amyloid cascade hypotheses. International Journal of Alzheimer's Disease, 2011, Article 276393.
8. Yokel, R. A. (2000). The toxicology of aluminum in the brain: A review. NeuroToxicology, 21(5), 813–828.
9. Exley, C. (2001). Aluminium and Alzheimer's disease: The science that describes the link. Amsterdam: Elsevier.

10. Krewski, D., Yokel, R. A., Nieboer, E., Borchelt, D., Cohen, J., Harry, J., ... & Rondeau, V. (2007). Aluminum and human health: A review. *Critical Reviews in Toxicology, 37*(5), 435–504.
11. Tomljenovic, L., & Shaw, C. A. (2011). Aluminum in the central nervous system (CNS): Toxicity in humans and animals, vaccine adjuvants, and autoimmunity. *Immunologic Research, 56*(2–3), 304–316.
12. FDA limit for aluminum in bottled water: U.S. Food and Drug Administration. (2020). *Bottled Water Everywhere: Keeping it Safe.*
13. WHO guideline for weekly aluminum intake: World Health Organization. (2011). Safety evaluation of certain food additives and contaminants: Prepared by the seventy-fourth meeting of the Joint FAO/WHO Expert Committee on Food Additives (JECFA). WHO Food Additives Series No. 64. Geneva, Switzerland: World Health Organization.
14. FDA limit for aluminum per vaccine dose: U.S. Food and Drug Administration. (2011). *Common ingredients in U.S. licensed vaccines.*
15. International Agency for Research on Cancer. (2012). *Formaldehyde.* In IARC monographs on the evaluation of carcinogenic risks to humans: Chemical agents and related occupations (Vol. 100F, pp. 401–435). Lyon, France: World Health Organization, International Agency for Research on Cancer.
16. Centers for Disease Control and Prevention (CDC). (2023). *Phenol: Emergency Response Card Information.* Agency for Toxic Substances and Disease Registry.
17. U.S. National Library of Medicine. (2021). *Phenol: Hazardous Substances Data Bank (HSDB).* PubChem Database.

18. International Programme on Chemical Safety (IPCS), World Health Organization (WHO). (1994). *Environmental Health Criteria 161: Phenol*. World Health Organization.
19. National Institute for Occupational Safety and Health (NIOSH). (2022). *NIOSH Pocket Guide to Chemical Hazards: Phenol*. Centers for Disease Control and Prevention.
20. European Medicines Agency. (2012). *Scientific discussion: Polysorbate 80*.
21. Cheng, S. H., et al. (2008). Polysorbate 80-modified nanoparticles for brain drug delivery: Preparation, characterization, and cytotoxicity. *International Journal of Pharmaceutics*, 350(1–2), 160–168.
22. Warren, R. S., & Lutz, R. J. (2011). Stability and characterization of polysorbate 80. In *Biopharmaceuticals: Biochemistry and Biotechnology* (2nd ed.). Wiley.
23. Sills, M. A., & Klein, L. J. (2005). Polysorbate 80-induced histamine release in humans. *Toxicology Letters*, 158(3), 219–223.
24. U.S. Food and Drug Administration. (2020). *Vaccine ingredients - Polysorbate 80*.
25. Chun, J. S., & Hartung, R. (1986). Effects of polysorbate 80 on the central nervous system of mice. *Toxicology and Applied Pharmacology*, 85(1), 89–98.
26. Sharp, P. M., & Hahn, B. H. (2011). Origins of HIV and the AIDS pandemic. *Cold Spring Harbor Perspectives in Medicine, 1*(1), a006841.
27. Institute of Medicine (US) Immunization Safety Review Committee. (2002). Immunization Safety Review: SV40 Contamination of Polio Vaccine and Cancer. National Academies Press (US).

28. Hayflick, L., & Moorhead, P. S. (1961). The serial cultivation of human diploid cell strains. *Experimental Cell Research, 25*(3), 585–621.
29. Jacobs, J. P., Jones, C. M., & Baille, J. P. (1970). Characteristics of a human diploid cell designated MRC-5. *Nature, 227*(5254), 168–170.
30. Wistar Institute. (n.d.). WI-38 Cell Line Legacy.
31. Schiffman, S. S., & Nagle, H. T. (2023). Sucralose metabolism and toxicity: A critical review. *Journal of Toxicology and Environmental Health, Part B: Critical Reviews, 26*(2), 41–61.

Chapter 7: Risks vs. Benefits

If you've ever raised a question about vaccine safety, chances are you've heard the age old response: *"The benefits outweigh the risks."* It's a phrase that gets repeated so often it almost feels like a default setting... quick, tidy, and meant to settle the conversation. But have you ever paused to ask: *What are the actual risks?* And *how exactly are they being weighed against the benefits?*

In this chapter, we're going to take a closer look at that very equation. We'll dive into the real, documented risks that come with vaccines. Risks that are often dismissed, downplayed, or misunderstood. We'll explore the science, the data, and even the fine print that many people never see. From known side effects to less acknowledged complications, we'll walk through the spectrum of what can go wrong, backed by research and real-world examples.

We'll also discuss the other side of the scale: the *benefits*. What are vaccines designed to protect against? How effective are they, and under what conditions? Are the outcomes as straightforward as we're often told?

By the end of this chapter, the goal isn't to tell you what to think. It's to give you the information you need to weigh both sides for yourself, with full context, not just catchphrases.

Let's start looking at the details behind the overused mantra: *"The benefits outweigh the risks."*

Before we get into the heart of the debate, comparing benefits and risks, we first need to pause and take a good look at what's actually being required. Too often, the vaccine conversation jumps straight to effectiveness or safety without ever acknowledging the sheer scope of what's on the table. Over the years, the recommended childhood vaccine schedule hasn't just grown... it's ballooned. What began as a short list of targeted suggestions has evolved into an extensive, rigidly enforced series of injections, now totaling over 70 doses by age 18. This isn't just about science anymore; it's about policy, momentum, and a phenomenon I like to call *requirement creep*. It's the quiet, incremental shift from occasional recommendations to unquestioned mandates. Before we can honestly weigh the pros and cons, we have to understand how we got here.

To understand just how dramatically things have changed, let's take a quick walk through the timeline.

In the early 20th century, the vaccine conversation centered almost entirely around smallpox. It was a single vaccine with a specific, well-defined purpose. Fast forward to the 1980s, and children were receiving around 22 recommended shots by the time they started school. But something shifted in the decades that followed. With the introduction of new vaccines and changes in policy, the number of required doses didn't just double, it multiplied. By the early 2000s, the CDC schedule had climbed to over 50 doses, and today, that number stands at more than 70 by age 18, with many given in the first few years of life. The expansion wasn't always accompanied by clear explanations or long-term safety studies, just new additions, year after year.

Understanding this evolution is essential, because the scale of what's required now dramatically changes the nature of the risk-benefit conversation. Let's dive into it.

The Vaccine Schedule - It All Started With One

In 1796, English physician Edward Jenner made an observation that laid the foundation for the future field of immunology. At the time, smallpox was considered a deadly and widespread disease causing immense suffering across Europe. However, Jenner noticed a curious pattern: milkmaids (young women who worked with cows) seemed to have a natural immunity. Many of these milkmaids had previously contracted cowpox, a much milder disease that caused pustules on the hands and arms but rarely led to serious illness or death.

Jenner hypothesized that exposure to cowpox somehow protected individuals from contracting the more severe smallpox. To test his theory, he conducted an experiment in May 1796 on an eight-year-old boy named James Phipps. Jenner took pus from the cowpox lesions on the hand of a milkmaid named Sarah Nelmes and introduced it into small cuts on Phipps' arm, a process known as inoculation. The boy developed mild symptoms of cowpox, like fever and local discomfort, but quickly recovered.

Several weeks later, Jenner exposed Phipps to pus from a smallpox lesion using a method known as *variolation*, which had been practiced previously to build resistance to smallpox. To Jenner's great success, Phipps did not develop smallpox, seeming to demonstrate that the cowpox inoculation had conferred protection. Jenner repeated this experiment on several other individuals, confirming that exposure to cowpox could safely and effectively prevent smallpox.

Although variolation, the practice of deliberately introducing smallpox material to build immunity, was already in use before Jenner, it carried significant risks because it involved actual smallpox virus, which could cause severe illness or death. Jenner's method of using cowpox was far safer. As this technique spread, a method of *arm-to-arm* transmission emerged, where material from the cowpox pustules of a recently innoculated individual was used to inoculate another person. Over time, this led to widespread acceptance and adoption of vaccination, a term coined from the Latin word *vacca*, meaning "cow," in honor of Jenner's work with cowpox.

Jenner's observations and innovations represented a turning point in medicine. His method eventually led to the development of the smallpox vaccine which some say led to the global eradication of smallpox in 1980, the first and only human disease to be eradicated.

Some researchers and independent thinkers however, suggested that the decline in smallpox mortality may not have been driven solely, or even primarily, by vaccination. Instead, they argue, there were likely multiple contributing factors. For instance, historical data shows that in several countries, smallpox deaths were already in sharp decline well before mass vaccination programs were introduced. This trend was especially noticeable in more developed nations, where improvements in sanitation, nutrition, and overall living conditions were already underway. These factors likely played a major role in reducing both the severity and the spread of the disease.

Another perspective centers on the idea of *natural* herd immunity. Over time, repeated natural exposure to smallpox helped build population-level immunity, particularly in densely populated areas where the disease had circulated for generations. Some even argue that the natural cycle of infection and immunity was disrupted, or at least altered, by vaccination, though not entirely replaced by it.

Adding to this discussion is the observation that in some parts of the world, smallpox disappeared even in areas with limited or poor access to vaccination. This raises an important question: if the vaccine was the only key to eradication, how did the disease vanish from places that lacked reliable vaccine infrastructure? Such inconsistencies suggest that other environmental or social factors might have also played a significant role in the decline of smallpox.

Fast forward to the 1940s, and the landscape of vaccination began to shift dramatically. Up until then, smallpox had been the primary, and in many cases the only, vaccine routinely recommended or administered. But almost overnight, that changed. Public health officials introduced a new combination vaccine known as DTP, designed to protect against three separate illnesses: diphtheria, tetanus, and pertussis (whooping cough). This "vaccine cocktail," as it's often called, delivered multiple immunizations in a single shot, and it marked a turning point in both medical strategy and public health policy.

With the introduction of DTP, the number of recommended vaccines for children suddenly quadrupled, from one to four, including smallpox. The change was swift and far-reaching. What had previously been a rare medical intervention now started to evolve into a standardized routine. The DTP vaccine was first licensed in 1948, and its widespread use ushered in an era where bundling vaccines into combination shots became common practice, both for convenience and compliance.

While the goal was to protect children from serious disease, this moment also marked the beginning of what can be called "requirement creep."

Once the precedent was set that multiple diseases could be targeted at once, via a single injection, the door opened wide for further additions. It wasn't just about safety anymore; it became about streamlining, scaling, and eventually mandating. This shift laid the groundwork for the modern vaccine schedule, which would continue to expand in both complexity and volume in the years to come.

Now, let's review our conversation about polio, the disease that struck fear into parents' hearts during the early to mid-1900s, and present how it became part of the requirement creep.

At the time, the image of children in iron lungs and braces became a powerful motivator for public health intervention. But as we've already discussed, the story of polio isn't quite as black and white as we were taught. While polio certainly did cause paralysis in some cases, most infections were actually mild or even asymptomatic. Many people who contracted polio never even knew they had it.

Still, the pressure to find a solution was immense. Enter Dr. Jonas Salk, who developed the first widely used polio vaccine in 1955. This vaccine used an inactivated (*killed*) version of the virus and was delivered by injection. A few years later, Albert Sabin introduced the oral polio vaccine (OPV), which used a *live*, attenuated virus and could be given on a sugar cube, much easier to administer to children en masse. Both versions were hailed as medical miracles, and quickly, the polio vaccine was added to the childhood immunization schedule.

By the late 1950s, what had started as a single smallpox shot just a few decades earlier had grown into a multi-vaccine routine. DTP (3 shots in one) was already in circulation, and now polio was joining the lineup. The vaccine schedule was starting to take shape; official, standardized, and widely promoted. And once again, what had been presented as a temporary, emergency measure began to solidify into a permanent public health policy. The focus had clearly shifted from individual, case-by-case recommendations to a one-size-fits-all mandate, with little room left for natural immunity or alternative approaches.

As we step into the 1960s and early 1970s, the vaccine train doesn't slow down. In fact, it picks up speed. By now, the idea of combining multiple vaccines into a single shot had caught on, and the next big "cocktail" to hit the scene was MMR: Measles, Mumps, and Rubella. Each one was marketed as a necessary defense against disease, and together, they were touted as another major step forward in modern medicine. But once again, if you peel back the layers, the story isn't quite as straightforward as the glossy pamphlets would have you believe.

Let's start with measles, which we've already touched on. Before the vaccine was introduced in 1963, measles was indeed a very common childhood illness, but for the vast majority of healthy children, it was more of a rite of passage than a medical emergency. Mortality rates had already dropped by more than 98% due to better nutrition, sanitation, and living standards, long before the vaccine ever made its debut. So while the vaccine may have contributed to reducing cases, the worst part of the disease was already fading.

Then there's mumps. Ask anyone over 50 and they'll probably recall having it as a kid. Swollen cheeks, sure. Maybe a few days home from school. But serious complications? Extremely rare. Mumps was another one of those common illnesses that gave you lifelong immunity and typically resolved on its own. The irony? Today, we vaccinate for mumps multiple times, and still have outbreaks... mostly among the fully vaccinated. But hey, just add another booster, right?

And rubella, or "German measles," rounds out the cocktail. For children, rubella is incredibly mild—many don't even know they have it. The real concern was for pregnant women, as contracting rubella during early pregnancy could lead to congenital rubella syndrome (CRS), a serious complication for the unborn baby. But here's the twist: instead of focusing on identifying and protecting women of childbearing age, the solution became mass vaccination of all children, boys and girls, regardless of individual risk. Another blanket policy for a very specific concern.

Here's where it gets paradoxical. The vaccine was administered broadly to *young children,* including girls long before they reached reproductive maturity. The idea was to reduce circulation of the virus in the population overall, thereby protecting everyone, including pregnant women. But there was a catch. The immunity provided by the vaccine is not lifelong. It's artificial active immunity, and unlike natural infection, it *wanes over time.*

So, here's the irony: if a young girl got vaccinated and never caught Rubella naturally, she was protected for only a short while… but by the time she reached adulthood, that protection faded. Natural active immunity was thwarted, and without natural immunity, she would actually be *more* vulnerable to Rubella during the exact time of life when it was most dangerous… during pregnancy. In essence, a policy designed to protect future mothers had inadvertently **increased** the risk by interrupting the natural cycle of immunity. It's a classic example of how short-term thinking in public health, can lead to unintended long-term consequences.

So by the end of the 1960s, the childhood vaccine schedule had quietly expanded to include a total of 9 doses: one smallpox, three from the DTP cocktail, three from the new MMR cocktail, and two doses of polio. What began just a few decades earlier as a single smallpox shot had evolved into a growing list of routine inoculations, administered not just when necessary, but now as a universal requirement. With each passing decade, the goalposts kept shifting, and the idea of personal choice or individualized risk assessment slowly faded from view.

By 1985, something dramatic had happened to the childhood vaccine schedule, it had *exploded*. What once began as a single smallpox vaccine decades earlier had now snowballed into a total of *23 recommended doses* for every child by the age of four. Let that number sink in for a second: twenty-three doses, most of them crammed into those tender early years when a child's immune system is still developing.

So how did we get here? The big jump wasn't just because of *new* vaccines being added, it was because of multiple doses of the same vaccines, administered over and over at short intervals. By two months old, babies were already being jabbed with Diphtheria, Tetanus, Pertussis, and Polio vaccines. Then at four months? The exact same round. And again at six months. The schedule repeated like a skipping record: another wave at 18 months, and then again at 48 months (four years old). That's *five doses each* of some vaccines by the time a child blows out their fourth birthday candles.

Add to that the now-standard MMR cocktail (Measles, Mumps, and Rubella) given around 12 months of age, and you've got three more vaccines right there. And just when it seemed the list couldn't grow longer, a new player joined the mix: the Hib vaccine, short for *Haemophilus influenzae type b*.

Hib might sound like the flu, but it's actually a different microbe entirely. One that may cause serious infections like meningitis and pneumonia, especially in young children. But here's the catch: prior to the vaccine's introduction, serious Hib disease had already been declining, and most healthy children who caught it recovered fully. Still, in 1985, a single dose of the Hib vaccine was added to the already-crowded schedule. This was the early version, the polysaccharide Hib vaccine, which wasn't very effective in babies under 18 months. But it was a stepping stone, and more versions would follow.

So by 1985, the reality was clear: we had gone from a single recommended vaccine in the early 1900s to a full-blown medical routine of *over twenty doses* in just the first few years of life. The logic, we were told, was that more doses meant more protection. But from the outside, it began to look like a system with a mind of its own. Growing in complexity and quantity, almost on autopilot.

It sets the stage perfectly for what's coming next: how the 1990s and beyond would continue this trend, introducing even more vaccines and further expanding the multi-dose strategy, while raising important questions about risk, benefit, and necessity.

By 1995, the vaccine schedule had crept forward yet again , and this time it welcomed another full-fledged member into the childhood lineup: Hepatitis B. Now, if you're thinking, *"Wait, isn't Hepatitis B mostly transmitted through needles and sex?"* You're exactly right. Hepatitis B is primarily passed between IV drug users, promiscuous sexual contact, or from mother to baby at birth. It's not a playground disease, and it's certainly not something your average onesie-wearing toddler is likely to pick up at daycare.

The justification for injecting every baby with a three-dose series of this vaccine (starting literally at birth) is rooted in the idea that *some* mothers might carry the virus and not know it. But routine screening of pregnant women for Hep B had already become a standard prenatal practice. So, if a mother tests negative, and the newborn is at virtually zero behavioral risk, it makes the universal Hep B vaccination feel a bit like using a fire hose to water a potted plant. *Three times!*

To make matters more bloated, this same decade introduced a new version of the Hib vaccine (Conjugate), which now required 4 doses. One each at 2, 4, and 6 months, followed by a booster at 12–15 months. That's three more shots, on top of the three doses of Hep B, making it six additional injections squeezed into the earliest, most developmentally delicate phase of life… all within just 10 years.

And mind you, this doesn't even count any optional flu shots.

So here we are: by the mid-90s, the schedule was expanding not because kids were getting sicker, but because the system kept finding new things to inject, often prophylactically, against diseases many kids were never likely to encounter in the first place. What started out as a focused public health effort was beginning to look more like a quota.

By 1996, another vaccine was added to the growing list of childhood "requirements": the Varicella Zoster vaccine, designed to prevent chickenpox. Now, if you're old enough to remember the 1980s or earlier, you probably remember "chickenpox parties". Seriously. We used to have gatherings where kids would play, share lollipops, and intentionally pass around the virus. Why? Because chickenpox was considered a mild, normal part of childhood… itchy and annoying, sure, but also a rite of passage that came with something invaluable: *natural, lifelong immunity.* And the younger the child was when they got it, the milder the illness tended to be. So when parents heard that another family's child had chickenpox, they'd often want their own young kids to be exposed as soon as possible.

But in '96, that tradition got a pharmaceutical overhaul. The chickenpox vaccine was introduced as a single-dose injection (later revised to two doses, but we'll get to that). Its goal? To provide artificial active immunity. The catch? Unlike the natural kind, this vaccine-induced protection is temporary. Immunity wanes over time, and rather than eliminating chickenpox, it may have just kicked the can down the road into adulthood, where things get riskier.

Here's the irony: adults who never experienced chickenpox as kids are more vulnerable to it later in life, and that's where shingles (a painful, blistering condition initiated by the varicella virus) enters the picture. Since the introduction of the chickenpox vaccine, shingles rates have surged, especially in younger adults. Why? Because natural infection previously would periodically "boost" the immune system's memory of the virus. But with less circulating wild virus, thanks to mass vaccination, those natural immune boosts disappeared, and shingles crept in to fill the gap.

In 1996, the vaccine was introduced as a single dose, typically given at 12–15 months of age. That brings the total number of recommended doses on the childhood vaccine schedule (from birth to age 6) to 28 doses, just 11 years after the 1985 schedule listed 23. And that's without even adding in the flu shot, which was about to make its grand entrance into the childhood lineup just a few years later.

So once again, what was once a temporary rash and a few missed school days has now become a reason to medicate the entire population, potentially creating more long-term complications than the original disease ever did.

Just when you thought the vaccine schedule couldn't get more crowded, along came 1998, bringing with it yet another addition: the rotavirus vaccine. This one was aimed at preventing a common viral infection that causes diarrhea in infants and young children. Now, to be fair, rotavirus can be miserable. Lots of diapers, some dehydration, and a few scary ER visits in the most severe cases. But for most healthy kids, it's just another short-lived childhood bug.

Despite that, the solution was — you guessed it — another vaccine. The first version of the rotavirus vaccine introduced in 1998 (RotaShield) required *three doses*. However, not long after its debut, it was pulled from the market due to safety concerns (sound familiar?), specifically its link to intussusception, a serious type of bowel obstruction in infants. Yikes! But don't worry, it didn't disappear for long. Newer versions came along just a few years later, and rotavirus remained part of the ever-growing lineup.

By this point in the late '90s, the total number of recommended vaccine doses before the age of 18 had climbed dramatically. Adding rotavirus to the list, along with the continued multi-dose requirements of hepatitis B, Hib, MMR, DTaP, polio, and now varicella, brought the total to *33 doses* by 1998. And keep in mind, this tally still doesn't even count annual flu shots, which were becoming more widely encouraged during this period.

What started as one smallpox jab back in the 1800s had now snowballed into a full-on vaccine marathon by age six. And the finish line? Well, it kept moving.

By the year 2000, the vaccine schedule had begun to feel like a game of vaccine musical chairs. One in, one out, and another one sliding into place. The rotavirus vaccine, which had just been introduced two years earlier, was removed from the schedule. Why? Intussusception. And just like that, three doses were subtracted from the official list. A rare moment of subtraction in a world of constant addition.

But of course, it wasn't long before a new vaccine was ready to take its place — enter *Hepatitis A.*

This one was designed to protect against a virus that causes temporary liver inflammation, usually spread through contaminated food or water. Think undercooked shellfish or that sketchy roadside taco stand. For most healthy kids, Hep A symptoms are mild and often go unnoticed. Maybe a low-grade fever, a little fatigue, along with some stomach discomfort. Honestly, most children bounce back without even realizing they were sick. But now, every child was scheduled to get two doses of the Hepatitis A vaccine, typically starting between 12 and 23 months of age, with the second dose six months later.

And while rotavirus was technically off the books for now, the rest of the vaccine lineup hadn't slowed down one bit. Kids were still getting multiple rounds of DTaP, polio, MMR, Hib, varicella, and hepatitis B… each with their own multi-dose regimens. Add in two new doses for Hep A, and by the year 2000, we were right back up to 32 recommended doses by age 18.

So even when a vaccine gets pulled for safety concerns, there's always another waiting in the wings to take its place, as if the goal was never to lighten the load, just to keep the conveyor belt running.

By 2004, the vaccine schedule officially entered the realm of "we're going to need a spreadsheet for this."

That year, the CDC formally added the flu vaccine to the routine childhood immunization schedule, recommending it annually for children aged 6–23 months. Yep, we've now crossed into *yearly vaccines*. And this wasn't a one-and-done shot. From this point on, every child was expected to receive a flu shot every single year, adding up to 18 additional doses by age 18, depending on when the child started. And let's not forget that the flu vaccine changes from year to year, meaning it's an ever-evolving cocktail of viral strains, preservatives, and adjuvants... injected again, and again, and again.

But the expansion didn't stop there. Just two years later, in 2006, the schedule was padded yet again. This time with the addition of two more vaccines: meningococcal and pneumococcal.

The meningococcal vaccine (MCV4) was introduced to protect against *Neisseria meningitidis*, a bacterium that can cause severe infections like meningitis and blood poisoning (sepsis). Serious stuff, to be sure, but still incredibly rare, especially in infants and young children. Nonetheless, one dose was now recommended around age 11–12, with a booster later in the teen years, for a total of 2 doses.

At the same time, the pneumococcal conjugate vaccine (PCV7) entered the scene to combat *Streptococcus pneumoniae*, which can cause pneumonia, ear infections, and in rare cases, meningitis or sepsis.

The CDC recommended 4 doses for all children — typically at 2, 4, 6, and 12–15 months.

Let's pause and do the math.

By 2006, a fully vaccinated child would have received:

- 3 doses of Hep B
- 5 doses of DTaP
- 4 doses of Hib
- 4 doses of IPV (polio)

- 2 doses of MMR
- 2 doses of Varicella
- 2 doses of Hep A
- 4 doses of PCV
- 2 doses of Meningococcal
- 1 flu shot every year, starting at 6 months, which by 18 years old could mean up to 18 flu shots

That brings us to a staggering *46 doses* by age 18, not even counting any additional boosters or catch-up shots. Just let that sink in for a moment.

And remember: these aren't just simple saline injections. Each dose includes multiple pathogenic antigens (many of which are bundled into combo "cocktail" shots), along with aluminum adjuvants, mercury (thimerosal), formaldehyde, polysorbate 80, antibiotics, yeast proteins, and trace amounts of viral, bacterial, human and multi species DNA, among other ingredients. With every added vaccine and every added dose, these toxic components are cumulatively injected into small, developing infant and child bodies, starting at birth, before a child even opens their eyes to the world.

So by 2006, the schedule wasn't just a list, it was a full-blown pharmaccutical roadmap, complete with increasingly complex timing, overlapping doses, and growing chemical exposure. And we're still not done!

Ah yes, 2007. The year the vaccine schedule officially seemed to say, *"We're just getting started."*

First, Rotavirus made its triumphant return, despite being pulled from the schedule just seven years earlier due to safety concerns. Remember the 2000 withdrawal because of *intussusception*, a type of bowel obstruction that was showing up in vaccinated infants? Well, apparently a new version of the vaccine, RotaTeq, was *"improved"* enough to be reintroduced. Instead of one dose like its predecessor, this time around the recommendation was for three oral doses, administered at 2, 4, and 6 months of age. So, the vaccine that was previously deemed too risky got a second chance. This time, babies were expected to swallow it three times.

But the bigger headline that year? The debut of the HPV vaccine.

Human papillomavirus (HPV) is a sexually transmitted infection linked to cervical cancer, as well as some other less common cancers. In 2007, the Gardasil vaccine was added to the schedule, originally for girls aged 11–12, with a 3-dose series spaced out over several months. And just like that, we were vaccinating preteens (who were still years away from sexual activity) with a fast-tracked vaccine that had never been tested against an inert placebo (more on that in a moment).

Gardasil was marketed as a breakthrough. "Protect your daughters (and later, your sons) from cervical cancer with just three simple injections". But like many things that seem too good to be true, the shine began to wear off, and questions started bubbling to the surface.

First, safety concerns. Within just a few years of its rollout, thousands of reports poured into the Vaccine Adverse Event Reporting System (VAERS), documenting everything from fainting spells and seizures to autoimmune reactions, premature ovarian failure, and even sudden deaths in previously healthy adolescents. These weren't fringe anecdotes whispered in obscure corners of the internet. They were real, documented cases, enough to prompt investigations in several countries and cause some nations (like Japan) to suspend active recommendations for the vaccine altogether.

And yet, public health agencies in the U.S. have largely dismissed these concerns as "coincidences" or statistical anomalies, insisting that the vaccine is "safe and effective." Critics argue that this conclusion is based on flawed trials and limited follow-up data, and — here we are again — no saline-based placebo was used in the original safety trials. Instead, the so-called "placebo" group was given an aluminum-containing adjuvant, the same immune-activating ingredient used in the vaccine itself. In other words, any adverse effects that could be caused by the aluminum wouldn't show up as a red flag, they'd appear in *both* groups, effectively masking potential safety signals.

Then there's the issue of necessity. HPV is very common, yes. But in most people, it clears on its own without causing any problems.

Cervical cancer, while serious, is already highly preventable through regular screening and Pap smears, especially in countries with modern healthcare systems. So vaccinating millions of children — including boys, who have no risk of cervical cancer (boys don't have cervixes), has prompted many to ask: Are we creating more risk than we're preventing?

And finally, the messaging. Parents are told that if they don't vaccinate their child with Gardasil, they're putting them at risk for cancer. No mention of side effects, no acknowledgement of controversy, no informed debate. Just a blanket of reassurance wrapped around a shot that's sparked lawsuits, injuries, and a growing number of families who are now raising their voices to say, *"We wish we had known more before we said yes."*

So here we are. A vaccine touted as a modern miracle, yet surrounded by a cloud of unanswered questions, conflicts of interest, and aggressive marketing tactics that leave little room for genuine informed consent.

So let's update our tally.

As of 2007, a child fully adhering to the CDC's recommended immunization schedule would receive:

- 3 doses of Hepatitis B
- 5 doses of DTaP (Diphtheria, Tetanus, Pertussis)
- 4 doses of Hib
- 4 doses of IPV (Polio)
- 2 doses of MMR
- 2 doses of Varicella (chickenpox)
- 2 doses of Hepatitis A
- 4 doses of Pneumococcal (PCV)
- 3 doses of Rotavirus (new version)

- 2 doses of Meningococcal
- Up to 18 doses of Influenza (1 per year from 6 months to 18 years)
- 3 doses of HPV (for adolescent girls in 2007, expanded to boys in later years)

That brings the new running total to at least 57 doses by age 18!

And here's where it gets more concerning: despite this dramatic rise in the number of vaccines, and the ever-increasing complexity of the schedule, remember, none of these vaccines have undergone saline-based, double-blind, placebo-controlled safety trials. Not one.

Reviewing from our discussion in chapter 6, in pharmaceutical research, the gold standard of testing is the double-blind, placebo-controlled trial, where one group receives the actual product, and the other receives an inert placebo, like saline. But when it comes to vaccines? That standard is astonishingly absent.

So, as the schedule bloats with more doses, more combinations, and more assumptions, we still lack the most basic standard of scientific evidence that should be a prerequisite when injecting substances into healthy infants and children... some before they've even left the hospital bassinet.

And yes, the schedule keeps growing...

Let's keep going on this little stroll through the maniacal vaccine schedule history, shall we? By the time we hit 2016, the vaccine count hadn't just grown, it had morphed into something far more intricate and, frankly, overwhelming. What started as a handful of shots to fend off a few serious diseases had now turned into a pharmaceutical to-do list that most parents could barely keep up with.

In 2016, kids were recommended to get around 54–56 doses by the time they hit 18. And remember, we're not just talking about more diseases, this was mostly due to more booster shots, combo vaccines, and, of course, the beloved annual flu shot. The HPV vaccine was now being pushed for both girls and boys, even though boys don't have cervixes—but hey, marketing knows no bounds, right?

So here we are in 2016, staring down a schedule with almost *five dozen injections*, all before graduation. Lovely.

Fast forward to 2020, and we're up to around 56 to 60 doses. Nothing major had been added yet in terms of *new* diseases, just the same old schedule beefed up with more boosters, more catch-ups, and increasingly aggressive school compliance policies.

It's also worth noting that by now, most of these shots are given during the *first four years of life,* a time when kids are still figuring out how to walk, talk, and—oh, you know—grow an immune system. Still think this schedule is a gentle recommendation? Try opting out and see how long before they threaten to kick your kid out of school.

Then came 2023, and with it, the official incorporation of the COVID-19 shot into the childhood immunization schedule. Yep, they made it routine. As in, "Your baby just turned six months? Great! Time for their mRNA dose!"

Depending on the product and age, kids could now receive three or more COVID shots on top of everything else. Combine that with annual flu vaccines, HPV doses, multiple boosters, and you're looking at **72+ injections** by the time a child turns 18.

Let that number sink in. Seventy-two!

So Where Are We Now?

What once started as a few targeted vaccines has ballooned into a lifelong pharmaceutical regimen. And no, this isn't about "a shot here and there." It's about repeated exposure to antigens, preservatives, adjuvants, and a whole cocktail of ingredients, often during the most fragile phases of development.

So, what's next? A monthly booster subscription plan?!

Now that you're aware of the sheer magnitude of what's actually being injected, layer upon layer of pathogenic antigens, toxic additives, and genetically engineered biological material, into the tiniest, most vulnerable humans in our population, it's time to address the big question: Is it worth it?

Let's talk about the benefits vs. risks.

Benefits

Okay, Let's have it. What are the benefits of this monstrously large vaccine schedule? Well, here it is:

On the benefit side, the argument is surprisingly short. In fact, it fits into one single, underwhelming paragraph.

Vaccines offer the *potential* for temporary, artificial, active immunity. That's it. That's the big payoff. No guarantees. No lifetime protection. No promises that you won't still contract or transmit the illness. Just a *chance*. A maybe, that your immune system might respond in a way that offers short-term resistance to a particular strain of a particular disease. (Just ask your doctor or any health official if vaccinations "guarantee immunity", and they will undoubtedly tell you "no".) And in many cases, any "immunity" you might get wears off, requiring additional boosters... indefinitely.

So that's it! That's the full extent of the benefit. We might *possibly* dodge an illness for a while.

Now buckle up, because the risk side of the equation is going to take a bit longer to unpack. Let's start peeling back those layers.

Risks

So, if the benefit of vaccination is a potential, temporary, artificial immunity, what exactly are we risking in return?

This is where the conversation gets real. Unlike the benefits, which are speculative and short-lived, the risks are *very real*, *very documented*, and in many cases, *very permanent*.

Before I get into specifics, let's begin with some basic categories, so we can begin to grasp just how deep this goes.

1. Biological Risks

Your child's immune system is an incredibly complex, intelligent system that's still developing in those early years. It's designed to encounter antigens naturally, through breathing, eating, touching, and living in the real world. But vaccination bypasses all of that.

When we inject multiple pathogens directly into the tissues and bloodstream, along with chemical adjuvants to "stimulate" a response, we bypass every natural line of defense. The immune system isn't primed to respond like that, especially not in infants. This immune overload can dysregulate normal function, setting the stage for autoimmune conditions like Type 1 diabetes, juvenile arthritis, and food allergies, just to name a few. It's not a mystery why childhood autoimmune diseases have skyrocketed in parallel with the vaccine schedule.[7,8,9,10,11]

2. Neurological Risks

Let's talk about the brain. Because guess what else is rapidly developing during those first two years of life? That's right, the central nervous system. So when vaccines contain known neurotoxins like mercury, aluminum and formaldehyde, we have a real problem. Aluminum, used in many vaccines as an adjuvant, crosses the blood-brain barrier and accumulates in brain tissue. Numerous studies and clinical reports have associated early exposure to aluminum with neurodevelopmental delays, speech regression, behavioral disorders, and yes, autism spectrum conditions. Even if the "autism debate" has been dismissed by mainstream media, the science surrounding neuroinflammation and mitochondrial dysfunction related to vaccine adjuvants is far from settled.[12,13,14,15,16,17]

Oh and remember, these ingredients aren't just injected once. We're talking about dozens of doses, in tight clusters, starting at just hours after birth.

3. Long-Term Health Consequences

We now live in an age where it's become "normal" for kids to carry EpiPens, have daily inhalers, and be on medications for anxiety and attention disorders before they even hit double digits. Childhood chronic illness is no longer rare, it's the expectation. Could this be connected to the simultaneous explosion of the vaccine schedule?

That's the million-dollar question.

Asthma, allergies, eczema, ADHD, and learning disorders have all risen dramatically in the last 40 years. Some of these shifts parallel the increases in specific vaccine exposures, such as aluminum, polysorbate 80, and thimerosal.

And don't forget the explosion of gastrointestinal issues and autoimmune gut disorders in children. The gut-brain connection is well established, and vaccines (by provoking inflammation and altering microbiota) can be a major disruptor to that delicate balance.

4. Genetic and Epigenetic Disruption

Emerging science is beginning to examine how vaccine components may impact gene expression. This isn't science fiction. Researchers are looking closely at how inflammation, adjuvants, and foreign DNA fragments (yes, human and animal DNA in vaccines) might trigger changes in how our genes express themselves, especially in young children whose systems are highly moldable.

Some scientists are asking: Are we creating epigenetic vulnerabilities that will echo through future generations?

5. Contamination and Unknowns

Vaccines aren't sterile in the way people assume. SV40, a cancer-causing virus, was famously discovered in the polio vaccine of the 1950s and 60s. More recently, DNA fragments from aborted fetal cell lines and retroviral contaminants have been identified in various vaccines. These are not theoretical risks, they are documented. And they beg a very uncomfortable question: *What else might be in that syringe that we haven't discovered yet?*

We've just scratched the surface, but already the risk side is looking, well, substantial. And keep in mind, this isn't even a complete list.

Next, I'll go deeper into individual reactions, injury reports, VAERS data, and why these side effects are so frequently dismissed, ignored, or underreported. If you've ever wondered why parents say, *"my child was never the same after that shot,"* this is where things really start to make sense.

Let's kick off the deep dive into specific conditions with one that's not only well-known, but also frequently acknowledged in both medical literature *and* vaccine package inserts:

Guillain-Barré Syndrome

Guillain-Barré Syndrome (GBS) is a rare but serious autoimmune condition in which the body's immune system turns against the peripheral nervous system... the network of nerves outside the brain and spinal cord. It typically starts with *tingling* or *weakness in the legs*, which can rapidly progress to *muscle weakness, paralysis*, and in severe cases, *respiratory failure*. Yes, GBS can land a person in the ICU, hooked up to a ventilator. Recovery is possible, but it can take months or even years, and some people are left with permanent neurological damage.

So, it's dangerous. Dangerous because it strikes suddenly, progresses quickly, and can be life-threatening if not treated aggressively. There's no cure, only supportive therapies like IV immunoglobulin (IVIG) or plasma exchange to calm the immune system down. And here's the most unsettling part: we still don't know exactly what triggers it in most people. But one thing is consistently flagged across the board—vaccines.

The connection between GBS and vaccines isn't just speculation, it's printed in black and white on multiple vaccine package inserts and acknowledged by the CDC itself! GBS is believed to be triggered in some individuals by immune activation gone wrong. In other words, a vaccine, especially one loaded with neurotoxic excipients like aluminum, polysorbate 80, or viral fragments grown on foreign tissue, can potentially send the immune system into overdrive. And for a small percentage of people, that immune response mistakenly starts attacking their own nerves.

It's a tragic irony: a shot designed to prevent illness can, in fact, trigger something far more serious than the disease itself.

Let's go through just a few examples of vaccines that either:

- List GBS in their package insert
- Have studies showing a statistical association
- Have VAERS reports that include GBS following vaccination

Influenza (Flu) Vaccine

- FDA-approved flu vaccine inserts (including FluLaval, Fluzone, and Fluarix) all list Guillain-Barré Syndromeas a potential adverse reaction.

- The CDC acknowledges that the 1976 swine flu vaccine had a well-documented spike in GBS cases, about 1 in 100,000 recipients.
- VAERS continues to receive thousands of reports related to GBS after seasonal flu shots.

Meningococcal Vaccine

- The Menactra insert includes GBS under reported adverse events.
- The CDC has acknowledged an increased risk of GBS in adolescents within 6 weeks of receiving this vaccine.

HPV Vaccine (Gardasil)

- Multiple case reports and post-marketing studies have associated Gardasil with the onset of GBS.
- The package insert notes autoimmune and neurological disorders post-vaccination, although causality is downplayed.

COVID-19 Vaccines (as of emergency authorization use)

- Both Pfizer and Johnson & Johnson have had GBS listed in post-marketing surveillance data.
- In July 2021, the FDA added a warning to the Johnson & Johnson COVID-19 vaccine about a small possible increased risk of GBS.

Tetanus Toxoid-containing Vaccines (DTaP, Tdap)

- GBS is listed as a potential adverse event in Tdap vaccine inserts (like Boostrix).
- Several case reports in peer-reviewed journals have explored the association.

What VAERS Reports Show:

As of the most recent publicly available VAERS (Vaccine Adverse Event Reporting System) data, there are *thousands* of reports linking various vaccines to Guillain-Barré Syndrome. It's worth noting that VAERS is a passive surveillance system and widely acknowledged to be *underreported*. Some estimates suggest **less than 1%** of actual adverse events are submitted (more on this later).

When a condition as serious as GBS shows up repeatedly in government databases, scientific literature, and official vaccine documentation, it deserves more than a footnote or a shrugged-off disclaimer. The risk might be "rare," but if it's your child, your sibling, your spouse—or you—it's not rare at all. It's life-altering.

And this is just *one* of the potential risks on the table. Ready to look at the next one?

Encephalitis

Let's keep this train moving with another serious, though often brushed aside, condition that shows up again and again in the literature, on vaccine inserts, and in thousands of VAERS reports: *Encephalitis*.

Encephalitis is *inflammation of the brain*. Sounds bad? That's because it is. When your brain, your body's command center, is inflamed, all bets are off. Symptoms can include *severe headache, fever, confusion, seizures, loss of consciousness*, and in some cases, *permanent brain damage* or *death*. In children, especially infants, encephalitis can be devastating, disrupting neurological development and leaving lasting cognitive or motor disabilities.

The kicker? We know vaccines are designed to stimulate the immune system, but sometimes that stimulation doesn't stop at antibody production. It turns systemic, crosses the blood-brain barrier, and *triggers inflammation in the brain itself.* In plain English: the very system designed to "protect" the child can occasionally go haywire and start attacking their own brain tissue!

Encephalitis can be triggered by infections, sure. But it can also be caused by an overreaction of the immune system, often referred to as an autoimmune response. Enter: vaccines.

Vaccines are *not* sterile saline. They are a cocktail of antigens, preservatives, adjuvants (like aluminum), surfactants (like polysorbate 80), viral or bacterial genetic material, human and animal cell remnants. And all of that is injected directly into the body, often multiple times before a child can even speak. Polysorbate 80 and other compounds can *open up the blood-brain barrier*, potentially allowing other ingredients, including neurotoxic aluminum, to reach the brain.

Now combine that with a genetically predisposed immune system or a vulnerable infant, and you've got the perfect storm for neuroinflammation.

Let's talk straight. This isn't conspiracy theory; this is straight from the *manufacturers' own documentation and CDC awareness:*

MMR (Measles-Mumps-Rubella)

- The MMR package insert lists encephalitis and encephalopathy under post-marketing adverse events.
- The CDC acknowledges that 1 in 1,000 children who contract natural measles can develop encephalitis. What they don't say quite as loudly is that the MMR vaccine itself has been linked to *post-vaccine encephalitis.*
- VAERS contains hundreds of reports citing the MMR vaccine followed by symptoms consistent with encephalitis.

DTaP (Diphtheria, Tetanus, Pertussis)

- Several DTaP vaccine inserts list encephalopathy (a broad term for brain dysfunction which can include encephalitis) as a potential adverse effect.
- Infamously, *"brain swelling"* or neurological damage has been at the heart of several vaccine injury court settlements related to DTaP.

Influenza Vaccine

- Numerous case studies and VAERS reports connect the flu vaccine with encephalitis, particularly acute disseminated encephalomyelitis (ADEM), a condition characterized by brief but intense inflammation in the brain and spinal cord.

HPV Vaccine (Gardasil)

- Reports to VAERS and published case series have described *autoimmune encephalitis* developing after Gardasil administration, especially in adolescent girls.

COVID-19 Vaccines

- A surge of post-marketing surveillance reports has associated mRNA vaccines with neurological complications, including encephalitis, though many are still labeled "rare" or "unconfirmed."

VAERS Reporting

VAERS stands for "Vaccine Adverse Event Reporting System". Later in chapter 8, I'll be discussing this program in more detail. As for now, the most current VAERS data available, *thousands of encephalitis and encephalopathy cases* have been filed following various routine vaccinations. VAERS is *passive*, meaning it likely captures just a fraction of what actually happens in real life.

Now let's be clear, correlation doesn't prove causation. But deductive reasoning becomes very important here.

When a condition shows up *across multiple vaccine types*, *across multiple manufacturers*, and is recognized both in package inserts and by the CDC, and when it makes *biological sense* based on known ingredients (aluminum, polysorbate, viral matter), you don't need a white lab coat to say: *this might not be as rare as they say.*

So, if a child got encephalitis from a toy, or a snack, or a pet, it would be front-page news and likely banned overnight. But when it's caused by a government-recommended, liability-free medical product? Suddenly it's a "rare coincidence." And we just move on.

But we're not moving on! We're moving forward, to the next risk in this long and growing list. The next topic is one that hits particularly close to home for many people:

Alzheimer's Disease

Now, I know what you might be thinking: *"Wait a second, Alzheimer's is a condition of the elderly. How does that connect to childhood vaccines?"*

Great question. Let's unpack it, slowly and logically, in the same spirit of deductive thinking we've been using throughout this book.

We already know that Alzheimer's Disease is a progressive neurodegenerative condition, marked by *memory loss, cognitive decline, confusion*, and ultimately, *severe impairment of basic functions*. What causes it? Well, science has pointed to a few key suspects: chronic inflammation in the brain, buildup of amyloid plaques, and wait for it… heavy metal toxicity, particularly aluminum and mercury. Both are well-documented neurotoxins. Both have been used in vaccines. And both have been detected in the brains of individuals suffering from Alzheimer's Disease.

The Aluminum Piece

Now, pause for a moment and consider: where do people get exposed to aluminum? It's not just in soda cans or cookware. In fact, one of the most direct and efficient ways aluminum enters the human body, bypassing the skin, the lungs, and the digestive system, is through injection. And guess what product is injected dozens of times into people from infancy through adulthood, many of which contain aluminum as an adjuvant? That's right—vaccines.

Aluminum salts (like aluminum hydroxide and aluminum phosphate) are included in many vaccines specifically to *provoke a stronger immune response.* But here's the problem: aluminum doesn't just disappear. Studies, yes even NIH-backed studies, have shown that *aluminum can accumulate in the brain*, particularly in regions involved in memory and cognition.

One groundbreaking study published in *Frontiers in Neurology* in 2018 by Dr. Christopher Exley (a leading authority on aluminum toxicity) examined brain tissue from individuals with Alzheimer's. What did he find? Sky-high levels of aluminum! Levels significantly higher than what's typically found in healthy brains.[56]

Add to that the NIH research suggesting chronic neuroinflammation is a key factor in Alzheimer's, and now you have to wonder: if we're injecting substances that both inflame the immune system and introduce neurotoxic metals into circulation, isn't it reasonable to ask whether this could contribute to or accelerate neurodegenerative processes?

And Now: Mercury

Mercury, specifically in the form of *thimerosal*, has long been used as a preservative in multi-dose vials of vaccines. Public health agencies insist it's safe in "trace amounts," but here's where the logic breaks down: *mercury is one of the most toxic substances known to the human nervous system.*

Even the tiniest amounts can cross the blood-brain barrier and accumulate in the cerebellum and hippocampus, two areas intimately tied to memory, learning, and coordination.

So why has it been used in vaccines for decades? Well, it was cheap, effective, and no one was demanding answers... until recently. While thimerosal has been phased out of most childhood vaccines in the U.S. (until 2025 some flu shots still contained it), millions of children were exposed in the 1980s, 90s, and early 2000s, precisely during a period when Alzheimer's rates (and neurological conditions in general) began to surge.

Add mercury's synergistic toxicity to aluminum—yes, research shows that when the two metals are combined, the neurological damage is exponentially worse—and you start to see how dangerous this cocktail really is.[55]

What Does This Have to Do with Kids?

It's easy to think, "Alzheimer's is for old people. Why should I care when we're talking about childhood vaccines?" But think deductively.

I often remind my patients: when it comes to your health, you've got to play the long game. Every choice you make (what you eat, how you move, what you put into your body) echoes into your future. Health isn't just about how you feel today; it's about setting the stage for how you'll function five, ten, even fifty years from now. Every decision leaves a footprint.

So, if neurotoxins are injected into a child, dozens of times from infancy through adolescence (and throughout adulthood), and those toxins accumulate in sensitive neural tissue, it's not unreasonable to suggest that these exposures are seeding neurological vulnerabilities— the kind that may not fully express themselves until decades later.

I'm not saying vaccines *cause* Alzheimer's directly. To say that would be to suggest that once injected, the patient would get the disease. However, if chronic brain inflammation, metal accumulation, and mitochondrial dysfunction are central features of the disease (and we're injecting substances known to cause those things) shouldn't we at least be asking the question: *"Could the accumulation of these known neurotoxins be contributing to the development of the disease"?*

And here's the real frustration. Despite growing concern, there are no long-term studies that track vaccinated vs. unvaccinated children into old age, looking at cognitive function or degenerative brain conditions. There are no randomized controlled trials evaluating aluminum or mercury exposure through vaccines over the full span of a human life.

If neurotoxin exposure is a known risk factor in brain degeneration, and if it's injected repeatedly into humans from infancy, *why is no one testing the long-term neurological impact of this practice?* Where are the decades-long safety studies on aluminum adjuvants in children? Spoiler: they don't exist.

And yet, we're told it's safe.

Trust the science?

How about we trust *reason*. And *logic*. And real-world *observations*. And above all, the courage to ask hard questions, even when they challenge authority.

In a world where Alzheimer's is now the 6th leading cause of death in the U.S., you'd think we'd want to understand every potential contributor. But instead of open investigation, we get dismissals, hand-waving, and vague reassurances.

Not here. Here, we're digging. We're reasoning. And we're moving forward... with eyes wide open.

Autism

Ah yes, *autism*. That one topic that everyone's afraid to talk about, especially if you dare utter the word "vaccines" in the same sentence. But let's not tiptoe around it. We're not here to win popularity contests; we're here to think logically, look at patterns, and ask questions that desperately need to be asked.

So let's talk about it.

Autism Spectrum Disorder (ASD) is a complex neurodevelopmental condition affecting communication, behavior, and social interaction. It's not a disease you "catch"—it's a condition that seems to be *developed*, often early in life, and once it's there, it's there for good.

And while there are many theories about what causes autism, genetics, environmental factors, gut health, you name it, the truth is: no one has definitively proven what causes it in every case. But here's the kicker… when something is labeled as "unknown," it leaves a big open door for honest inquiry. So let's walk through that door.

First, let's talk about timing. Ask parents of children with autism, and you'll hear many familiar stories: *"He was developing normally… then after a round of shots, everything changed."* That's not a conspiracy theory, that's a pattern. And it's a pattern that has shown up thousands upon thousands of times in personal stories, in case studies, in VAERS entries, and even in published studies[1,4,5,6].

One of the most talked-about studies in this space was in 1998, when Dr. Andrew Wakefield and 12 co-authors published a paper in *The Lancet* suggesting a potential link between the MMR (measles, mumps, rubella) vaccine and autism, based on a small case series of 12 children. Importantly, *the paper did not claim to prove causation,* but it did raise concerns and called for more research. The media, however, sensationalized the paper as proof that MMR causes autism, sparking a firestorm of controversy.

By 2010, The Lancet officially pulled the plug on the paper, and it was formally retracted. Around the same time, the UK's General Medical Council (GMC) had wrapped up a lengthy investigation into Andrew Wakefield. The fallout? His medical license was revoked.

So why do I refer to a paper that was officially retracted by the medical establishment and written by an author widely disgraced in the media? Simple. Because there's *more to the story* than you've been told. Or, as Paul Harvey would say, here's "the rest of the story."

Dr. Andrew Wakefield wasn't the only name on that infamous *Lancet* paper. There were 12 co-authors in total. Of them, 11 kept their medical licenses. One other doctor, Dr. John Walker-Smith, a senior pediatric gastroenterologist, was also struck off the UK medical register in 2010 based on similar allegations. But here's the part you probably didn't hear: in 2012, he appealed… and won.

Funny how you never hear that part in the headlines, right? The moment someone even mentions "vaccines" and "autism" in the same breath, critics jump straight to, "Wakefield was discredited!" But rarely does anyone mention that his senior co-author fought the same charges and was *fully vindicated* in court.

Let's take a moment to apply some simple logic.

You've probably heard of the old deductive reasoning formula called the *Transitive Property of Equality* which states: *If A equals B, and B equals C, then A equals C*. It's a tidy, rational way to arrive at a conclusion, and it fits perfectly when looking at what happened to Dr. Andrew Wakefield and his colleague, Dr. John Walker-Smith.

Both doctors were co-authors on the now-infamous 1998 *Lancet* paper that explored a possible connection between the MMR vaccine and autism in a group of children. That paper triggered a media firestorm and a long investigation by the UK's General Medical Council (GMC), which eventually stripped both men of their medical licenses in 2010 for alleged misconduct in how the study was conducted.

But here's where it gets interesting: Dr. John Walker-Smith appealed the decision. And in 2012, the UK High Court overturned the GMC's ruling, stating that their decision was "based on inadequate and superficial reasoning" and that Walker-Smith's license should be fully reinstated.

Now, the misconduct charges the GMC brought against Walker-Smith and Wakefield were largely based on the *same paper* and the *same data*. So logically speaking, if the court found that the GMC's judgment in Walker-Smith's case was flawed (and that paper is the exact one Wakefield was punished for, too) then shouldn't the core of the case against Wakefield be considered flawed as well?

In short: If Walker-Smith was exonerated based on the court's conclusion that the GMC acted improperly, and Wakefield was accused of the same research conduct, then it's entirely reasonable to argue that Wakefield deserves the same reconsideration.

But here's the catch: *Wakefield never had his day in court.* Whether he chose not to appeal, or wasn't given the same opportunity, the fact remains, and his case was never reviewed by the higher British authority like Walker-Smith's was.

So, Wakefield was not *legally* "vindicated." But based on simple logic and shared circumstances, there's a very strong case that at least part of the narrative used to discredit him was built on sand. You won't hear that part of the story from the media. But now... you know.

And as far as the claim of no correlation between autism and vaccines? While separate from the Wakefield controversy, it's worth noting that numerous families have received compensation through the U.S. National Vaccine Injury Compensation Program for children who developed autism-like symptoms after vaccination. That's a matter of public record.

So, even though the Lancet paper was retracted, and the media, medical community, and pharmaceutical industries continue to do their best to try to discredit Wakefield, let's be honest: it didn't spark the debate; it just exposed the crack in the dam.[1]

Since then, the tireless mantra has been "the science is settled." But is it? In 2014, a CDC whistleblower, Dr. William Thompson, came forward claiming that CDC researchers manipulated data in a 2004 study to hide a statistically significant connection between the MMR vaccine and autism in African American boys.[2] The response? Silence. Dismissal. And the media... crickets.

The Data That Was Never Meant to Be Found

When Robert F. Kennedy, Jr. stepped into his new role as Secretary of Health and Human Services in 2025, he didn't walk into the building with wide-eyed wonder, he walked in with a mission. For decades, he had challenged the very agencies he now commanded. He had sued them. Investigated them. Exposed them. And now he was their boss.

So what did he do with that newfound authority?

He opened the filing cabinets.

He pulled up the digital archives.

He started asking questions that, for years, no one in power dared to ask.

And that's when he found it.

Buried deep in the CDC's records, behind years of internal emails, statistical revisions, and quiet retractions, was a set of data that had once sent shockwaves through a team of CDC scientists back in the late 1990's. It was part of an early analysis of the Vaccine Safety Datalink (VSD), a government-run treasure trove of health records and vaccination data. The study, led by Dr. Thomas Verstraeten, had examined the possible effects of thimerosal, found in many vaccines at the time, including the Hepatitis B vaccine given to newborns.

The results? Alarming.

The original analysis showed that infant boys who received the Hep B vaccine within the first month of life were significantly more likely to develop autism than those who received it later. In some cases, as much as 2.5 to 3 times higher risk. The findings were so jarring that internal CDC memos used phrases like, *"We have a problem,"* and *"This will have to be handled carefully."*

And "handled" it was.

Over the course of the next three years, the CDC held a series of closed-door meetings. The data was massaged. Revisions were made. Models were re-run. And with each iteration, the statistical significance faded. By the time the final version of the study was published in *Pediatrics* in 2003, the message had been laundered clean: *"No consistent association."*

Case closed. At least publicly.

But internally, concern remained. And outside the CDC, independent researchers were picking up the scent. Studies by Gallagher and Goodman in 2008 showed that *boys who received all three Hepatitis B shots were up to three times more likely to be diagnosed with autism* or other developmental delays. Yet these findings, too, were shrugged off by mainstream media and medical authorities.

Fast forward to 2025.

Now, with the keys to the very agency that had buried the data, *Secretary Kennedy reviewed the original VSD files himself.* The evidence (the early emails, the draft studies, the internal contradictions) was all still there.

The only thing missing? Accountability.

"We've long suspected the data was there," Kennedy said. "Now I've seen it firsthand. This isn't just a question of bad science, it's a question of betrayed public trust. And our babies paid the price."

And just like that, a decades-old suspicion turned into a full-blown government reckoning. The study they tried to forget had come back, not through FOIA requests or whistleblower leaks, but through the determination of a man who had spent most of his career outside the system… and now stood at its head.

Let's Return to Ingredients

We already discussed aluminum and mercury in the context of Alzheimer's. But here's the hard truth: those same neurotoxic ingredients are being injected into infants and toddlers at the most critical stage of brain development.

Think about it: the human brain develops rapidly in the first few years of life. It's laying down neural pathways, forming synaptic connections, calibrating the immune system, and fine-tuning hormonal balances.

Now add to that:

- Thimerosal (ethylmercury): a known neurotoxin.
- Aluminum adjuvants: disrupt mitochondrial function and cause chronic inflammation.
- Polysorbate 80: known to open the blood-brain barrier, potentially allowing metals and pathogens to enter brain tissue.
- Formaldehyde: classified as a human carcinogen, used to "inactivate" viruses in vaccines.

These aren't benign substances. They're not things you'd stir into a toddler's breakfast. Yet they're injected into them dozens of times, at precisely the time when their brains are most vulnerable.

Now, Let's Talk Stats

In the 1970s, autism was virtually unheard of. The rate was approximately 1 in 10,000.

Today? As of 2023, the CDC reports that autism affects 1 in 36 children in the United States.[3 1 in 36! And in boys, that rate is even higher.

Now here's where things get interesting:

Look at how these numbers increased next to the increase in vaccine doses in the childhood vaccine schedule!

Year	Autism Rate	# of Vaccine Doses by Age 18
1970	1 in 10,000	9 doses
1985	1 in 2,500	23 doses
2000	1 in 150	36 doses
2023	1 in 36	74 doses

That's not just a coincidence. That's a correlation so strong it begs for honest investigation.

I know, I know, correlation isn't causation… but as the saying goes: when there's smoke, there's fire. At the very least, the public deserves transparency, robust safety trials, and long-term studies that compare one vaccinated group to another completely unvaccinated group. Let's be honest… this kind of research still hasn't happened. And why not? Because they already know what it would show!

A true, long-term study comparing vaccinated to completely unvaccinated people would blow the lid off the entire narrative. The results would almost certainly reveal what many of us have suspected for years: that unvaccinated individuals are, on average, healthier. Fewer chronic conditions. Fewer neurological issues. Fewer autoimmune problems. If that kind of data were made public, it would expose the flaws, maybe even the fraud, of the entire vaccination program. And they can't afford that. So instead of doing the research, they just keep repeating the mantra: "safe and effective." Over and over and over again. As if saying it enough times will make it true.

Now, if above table didn't already make you raise an eyebrow, let's go ahead and lay it out in graph form, because sometimes a picture really is worth a thousand data points. (Straight line is trend line)

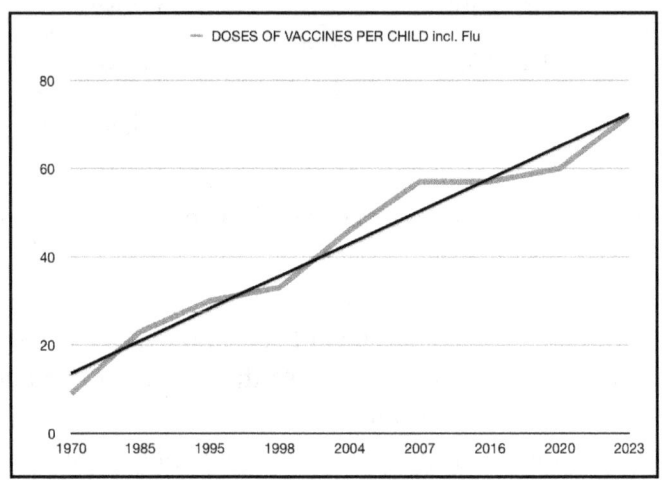

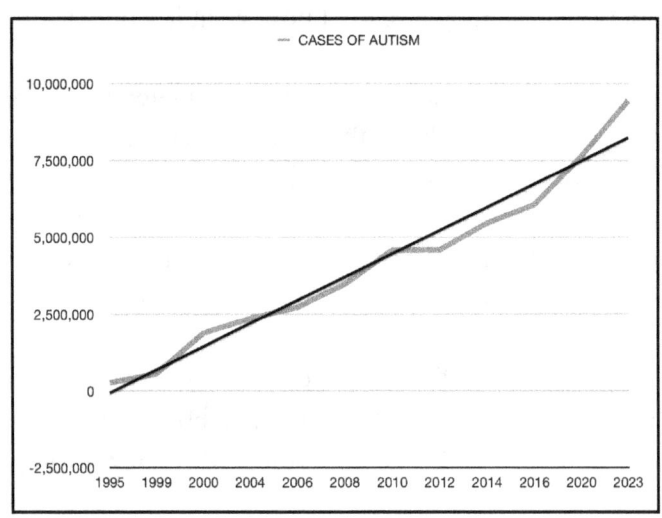

The first graph? That's the steadily climbing vaccine schedule we covered earlier in this chapter.

The second? That's the gut-punch rise in autism diagnoses over the past five decades.

Notice any similarities?! Now, of course, the usual suspects will smugly chime in with "correlation doesn't equal causation," like it's some kind of intellectual mic drop. But come on, do we really need a PhD in epidemiology to see the glaringly obvious parallel here?

Still not convinced? Look at them side by side.

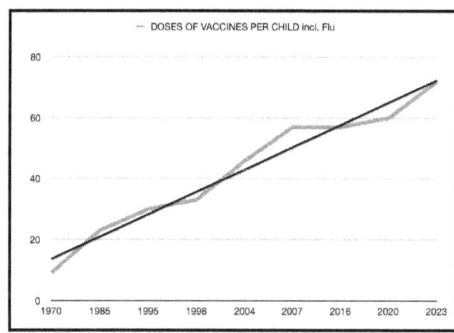 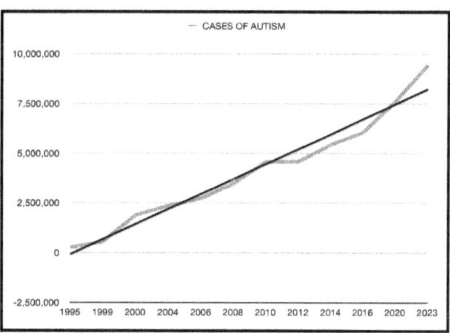

See the trend lines? You could overlay the two graphs and see that they climb together like synchronized swimmers.

Now I don't know about you, but if I were seeing this combined visual for the first time and genuinely wondering whether there could be even a *possibility* of a link between the explosion in vaccines and the explosion in autism... well, this would stop me dead in my tracks. You don't need a conspiracy theory when a graph slaps you in the face with common sense.

The Deductive Rationale

Let's break it down in logic terms:

- **Premise 1**: Aluminum, mercury, and other vaccine excipients are neurotoxic.
- **Premise 2**: These ingredients are injected into infants and toddlers during peak brain development.
- **Premise 3**: Autism is a neurological disorder that appears in early childhood.
- **Premise 4**: The rate of autism has risen in direct proportion to the increase in vaccine doses over the last 50 years.
- **Conclusion**: It is logically consistent, and medically responsible, to suspect that vaccines and their ingredients may play a contributing role in the rise of autism.

That's not conspiracy. That's deductive reasoning.

So… are vaccines the sole cause of autism? Probably not. But is it even slightly rational to pretend they have *nothing* to do with it?

That's the real insanity.

Parkinson's Disease

Let's talk about Parkinson's Disease.

When most people hear "Parkinson's," they think of tremors, shuffling gait, or maybe even celebrities like Michael J. Fox or athletes like Kirk Gibson. But there's a lot more to the story than just shaky hands. Parkinson's is a progressive neurodegenerative disorder, meaning it gets worse over time and primarily affects movement and coordination. It's marked by the loss of dopamine-producing neurons in a part of the brain called the substantia nigra. The result? Muscle rigidity, tremors, balance issues, and eventually, cognitive decline. But why are those brain cells dying?

Here's where it gets interesting, and deeply concerning.

A Quick History

Parkinson's was first described in 1817 by British physician James Parkinson. For over a century, it was considered rare. In fact, by mid-20th century (around the 1950s), Parkinson's was still a relatively uncommon diagnosis, affecting fewer than 1 in 10,000 people. Fast forward to today: Parkinson's now affects over 10 million people globally, and the rate in industrialized nations like the U.S. has skyrocketed. Recent estimates suggest incidence rates have more than doubled in the past few decades alone.

So the natural question becomes: *What changed?*

The NIH Admits It: Parkinson's Is Tied to Environmental Toxins

According to the National Institutes of Health (NIH),

> *"Many researchers now believe Parkinson's results from a combination of genetic and environmental factors, such as exposure to toxins."*[18]

Let that sink in. Not just genes. *Environmental toxins.*

So what are those toxins? Pesticides, heavy metals, industrial pollutants... and yes, ingredients found in vaccines.

This isn't conspiracy. It's logic, facts, and reason.

A Refresher on What's in the Syringe

In the last chapter, we talked about some of the most concerning ingredients in vaccines. Substances that are classified as neurotoxic, meaning they can damage the nervous system.

Here's a quick reminder:

- Mercury (Thimerosal) – Even in trace amounts, it accumulates in the brain and disrupts neural function.
- Aluminum salts (adjuvants) – Trigger chronic immune activation and are linked to neuroinflammation.
- Formaldehyde – A known carcinogen that also has neurotoxic potential.
- Polysorbate 80 – A chemical emulsifier that can cross the blood-brain barrier, potentially allowing other toxins in.

- Phenol / Phenoxyethanol – Used as preservatives, both have known toxic effects on the central nervous system.[27]

Individually, these substances raise red flags. But together (and especially when administered repeatedly) they form a *toxic cocktail.*

Now add in cumulative exposure over dozens of doses throughout childhood and adulthood. Is it any wonder we're seeing an explosion in neurodegenerative disorders?

Connect the Dots: Vaccination Schedules and Parkinson's Incidence

Let's look at the timelines.

In the 1950s, a child received roughly 4-5 vaccine doses total by age 6. Today? That number is closer to 72 doses by age 18 according to the CDC's current schedule. That's a 14-fold increase, not to mention the ongoing lifetime accumulation of booster shots!

Now let's compare that to Parkinson's trends. In 1976, the estimated global prevalence of Parkinson's was around 2 million people. As of 2024, it's well over 10 million. A fivefold increase! And studies project that number will double again by 2040.[19,20,21]

Coincidence?

We already know these ingredients are neurotoxic. We know they're injected (not inhaled or ingested) which bypasses normal detox pathways. We know the body doesn't always eliminate them efficiently, especially when they cross the blood-brain barrier. And now the NIH itself tells us that environmental toxins are a known factor in Parkinson's.

So if we follow the logic, the conclusion isn't just possible, it's probable.

Vaccines are not the only environmental factor involved in the Parkinson's epidemic, but to ignore them in this conversation is not only irresponsible, it's scientifically dishonest.

We question everything else in science. Why should this be off limits?

Let's talk about another brain-and-body disrupter…

Multiple Sclerosis.

MS is one of those diseases people hear about but rarely understand, until it hits someone close to home. And it's hitting more and more people.

Multiple Sclerosis is an autoimmune disease where the immune system mistakenly attacks the protective myelin sheath that covers nerve fibers in the brain and spinal cord. Think of myelin like the insulation on electrical wires. When that insulation breaks down, the messages traveling along the "wires" short-circuit. The result? Brain-body communication begins to fail. Literally.

What does MS look like? Symptoms can vary, but here's a sample menu:

- Muscle weakness or paralysis
- Fatigue that borders on debilitating
- Vision loss or double vision
- Numbness and tingling
- Balance and coordination issues
- Cognitive dysfunction

Over time, MS can lead to significant disability, like loss of mobility, speech, and independence. While not always fatal, it's progressive. And it has no known cure.

But here's the million-dollar question: *Why is this happening? Why is MS becoming more common?*

A Disease That Used to Be Rare

In the mid-20th century, Multiple Sclerosis was practically a medical curiosity. Estimated prevalence in the 1950s hovered around 20 cases per 100,000 people in the U.S.

Fast forward to today: prevalence has exploded. According to the National MS Society and global studies, the rate is now over 300 per 100,000 in some industrialized countries, including the U.S., Canada, and parts of Europe.[22,23,24,25,27] That's a 15-fold increase in about 70 years!

So what changed? Cue the same familiar suspects: environmental toxins, especially neurotoxins introduced through vaccination.

I hate to sound like a broken record, but let's bring back some of our greatest hits:

- Mercury (Thimerosal): A powerful neurotoxin that accumulates in brain tissue. It's been shown to impair mitochondrial function, damage oligodendrocytes (the cells that produce myelin), and provoke autoimmune reactivity, all of which line up perfectly with MS pathology.
- Aluminum (as adjuvants): Triggers chronic immune activation, can cross the blood-brain barrier, and has been linked to neuroinflammation. Again, all relevant in MS. One study even found aluminum deposits in the brain tissue of MS patients.
- Phenol / Phenoxyethanol: Common vaccine preservatives. These substances are known to affect cellular membranes and can act as central nervous system depressants and irritants.[27] Not exactly something you want swimming around your central nervous system.

Now imagine receiving dozens of doses containing *some or all* of these over your lifetime, starting when your brain and immune system are still developing.

The Timeline: Here We Go Again

Here's that uncomfortable but necessary comparison again.

- In the 1950s: U.S. children received around 4-5 total vaccine doses by school age.
- Today: It's over 70 doses by age 18, with many adults receiving boosters, flu shots, and now annual mRNA doses into old age.[28]

Meanwhile...

- In the 1950s: MS affected ~20 per 100,000 Americans.
- By 2024: That number exceeds 300 per 100,000 in many regions. That's a staggering 1,400% increase.

Coincidence?

Again, the official narrative loves to say "We don't know what causes MS." But then in the next breath, institutions like the National Institutes of Health and National MS Society admit that "genetic and environmental triggers" are likely to blame.

So here's a deductive question: If neurotoxins are *known* to damage myelin-producing cells, provoke autoimmunity, and inflame brain tissue... and if we've been injecting those same toxins directly into human tissue in escalating doses for decades... is it really that hard to connect the dots?

I'm not saying vaccines are the only factor in MS. But pretending they're not a major piece of the puzzle? That's not science. That's denial.

The Food Allergy Explosion

Let's take a moment to talk about something that didn't even exist a few generations ago: *"No peanuts allowed"* zones, epipens in every classroom, and parents terrified of cupcakes at birthday parties.

Peanut allergies. Egg allergies. Dairy allergies. Soy, wheat, gelatin. Things that kids used to eat without a second thought are now considered biohazards in elementary schools. And we're not just talking about an itchy rash here, these are *anaphylactic*, sometimes deadly, full-blown immune overreactions. So once again: What changed?

Spoiler alert: Kids didn't suddenly evolve to be allergic to everything. Something *external* is provoking this madness. And here's where the conversation gets very, very uncomfortable.

First, the Science of Allergies 101

An allergy is an immune system overreaction to something that should be harmless, like food proteins. Your immune system sees peanut, or milk, or egg protein, and instead of going, "Cool, we've seen this before," it goes DEFCON 1 and sends the immune troops in to nuke it from orbit. That reaction, especially when it includes histamine and mast cell activation, can become life-threatening in seconds.

So why does the body *decide* to react that way? Because it's been trained to. And this is where vaccines come in.

Vaccines are designed to train the immune system... sometimes too well! You see, vaccines work by exposing the body to an antigen (like a virus protein) along with an adjuvant which is a chemical designed to *supercharge the immune response.* Think of adjuvants like the drill sergeant screaming in the face of your immune cells, "PAY ATTENTION TO THIS!"

And they work. Too well, sometimes.

Now here's the kicker: vaccines don't just contain viral or bacterial particles and adjuvants. They also contain biological residue from how the vaccine was grown. That includes:

- Egg proteins (from chicken embryos)
- Cow serum (used in cell culture media)
- Peanut oil (used in vaccine emulsifiers and as excipients in past formulations)
- Gelatin (from pigs or cows)
- Yeast proteins
- Polysorbate 80, aluminum, and other adjuvants which make sure your immune system reacts... hard.

Let's make this really simple.

Eggs come from chickens. Vaccines are cultured in chicken embryos.
Milk comes from cows. Many vaccines are made using fetal bovine serum.
Peanuts come from—wait for it—peanuts. Peanut oil

derivatives have historically been used in vaccine emulsifiers and may still be present in trace, undisclosed amounts.

Soy? Gelatin? Yeast? All used in vaccine production.

Now imagine injecting these substances directly into the muscle tissue of a 2-month-old infant. Not once, but dozens of times. All while using an aluminum adjuvant that's literally designed to scream at the immune system to pay attention and *never forget what it sees.*

And then we wonder why the kid's immune system now treats pancakes like a terrorist attack.

We aren't just exposing children to food proteins, we're weaponizing them.

If a kid ate an egg, their digestive system would break it down and decide whether it was friend or foe in a calm, natural way. But when you inject egg protein into the body with aluminum, polysorbate 80, and phenol, you're telling the immune system: "THIS is a threat. Burn it down."

Do that enough times, and the immune system learns the lesson, forever. The body doesn't forget. That's how you get a first grader with an EpiPen strapped to their backpack for fear that a slice of birthday cake might shut down their airway.

We didn't evolve into this epidemic. *We engineered it.*

So if we're training the immune system to attack whatever is in the injection, and we inject it *again and again* from infancy into adulthood, is it really such a mystery that people start developing chronic, life-threatening reactions to the ingredients they've been injected with?

It's like we taught the immune system to react this way... because we did!

Let's go back 50–60 years.

In the 1950s and 60s, food allergies were rare. Like, weird rare. Your grandmother didn't check for peanut butter on the playground. There were no "nut-free" lunch tables.

Then, as vaccine schedules exploded, especially in the late '80s and '90s, so did food allergies. Consider:

- In 1960, the U.S. vaccine schedule included 4–5 total doses.
- In 2024, that number is over 70 doses by age 18.
- Meanwhile, childhood peanut allergies have tripled since the 1990s.
- Milk, egg, and soy allergies are also up dramatically. Some estimates say over 400% in the last 30 years.[32,36]
- Entire schools now carry epinephrine as standard protocol.

Let's spell it out: If you inject egg protein alongside an aluminum adjuvant, the body associates egg with a threat. Do it again. And again. Congratulations, you may have just trained the body to see eggs as a biochemical terrorist. Welcome to your new lifelong food allergy.

It's called *bystander sensitization.* And it's a documented immunological phenomenon. We've just chosen to ignore it when it doesn't serve the narrative.

But wait, there's more!

A 2002 paper in the *Journal of Allergy and Clinical Immunology* noted that vaccines could "lead to allergic sensitization to food proteins."[37] But instead of asking, "Wait, should we fix this?" they just moved on. Because again, questioning the vaccine program is career suicide in certain circles.

And here's the irony: They tell parents, "Feed your baby peanuts early to prevent allergies." But they also inject trace peanut protein into babies' muscle tissue before the gut immune system is even mature, and then trained the child's body to attack it. It's not that the body can't handle peanuts, it's that we taught it to panic when it sees them.

Let that sink in.

Now, let's talk about something no parent ever wants to see:

Seizures

Eyes roll back. Body jerks. Maybe there's foaming, confusion, unconsciousness. It's terrifying. And today? It's common.

And not just grand mal seizures. We're seeing absence seizures (where kids check out mid-sentence), myoclonic seizures (sudden jerks), febrile seizures, epileptic syndromes, and more. We even gave it a new name, "Seizure Spectrum Disorder", because apparently slapping "spectrum" on everything helps explain what we refuse to look at directly.

But here's the real shocker: seizure disorders have absolutely exploded over the last several decades. And once again, instead of asking *why*, we're just handing out anti-convulsants like candy.

So... what's happening inside these kids' brains?

Electricity doesn't just misfire for no reason. Seizures are caused by abnormal bursts of electrical activity in the brain. In healthy brains, neurons fire in an organized way. During a seizure, it's chaotic overdrive, like a lightning storm behind the eyes. This can be due to inflammation, toxicity, mitochondrial dysfunction, or disruption of neurotransmitters. All things that can be triggered or worsened by the known ingredients in vaccines.

Let's relate them to seizures:

- Aluminum is a potent immune stimulator that can cross the blood-brain barrier and trigger neuroinflammation.
- Mercury (Thimerosal) is one of the most well-documented neurotoxins in existence, known to disrupt neural function even in microgram amounts.
- Phenol and Phenoxyethanol, used as preservatives, can affect the central nervous system and lower the seizure threshold.

- Polysorbate 80 can act as a Trojan horse, pulling other toxins across the blood-brain barrier and into the most sensitive organ in the body, the developing brain.

Now combine these with an immature nervous system, rapidly developing brain tissue, and multiple injections in a compressed schedule. You don't need a medical degree to say, *"Yeah, this might cause some problems."*

The Timeline: More Doses, More Seizures

- In the 1950s and 60s, seizures in children were considered unusual medical events.
- By the 1980s, seizure reports started showing up in vaccine injury tables (including DTaP, MMR, and whole-cell pertussis vaccines).
- In 2024, seizure disorders are now one of the most common neurological issues in children, affecting 1 in 26 Americans across the lifespan, and many children begin showing signs before age 5.

Meanwhile, the vaccine schedule:

- 1950s: 4–5 doses by age 6.
- Today: 72 doses by age 18.

The math isn't complicated.

And here's the uncomfortable truth: seizures are a *known* adverse reaction to multiple vaccines. It's right there in the package inserts. In fact, for years, the federal Vaccine Injury Compensation Program (VICP) has paid out settlements for vaccine-induced seizure disorders, especially when they resulted in long-term damage or were followed by regression into autism.

So if we *know* these ingredients can inflame the brain… if we *know* seizures are a neurological symptom of inflammation or toxicity… and if we *know* that these events often occur within hours to days of routine vaccination… why are we still pretending that this is just "rare," "genetic," or "bad luck"?

At some point, refusing to connect the dots isn't just ignorance, it's negligence.

Tics and Tourette's

Let's zoom in on something that seems small—at first.

A blink. A sniff. A shoulder jerk. A grunt. Maybe even a word repeated compulsively.

These aren't just habits. These are *tics,* and when they cluster together and persist, we call it Tourette's Syndrome. It's a neurological disorder where the brain loses full control over motor and vocal impulses… and it's on the rise.

So what's going on? Are we just "noticing it more"? Or is something provoking the brain into these glitches?

What Are Tics and Tourette's, Really?

Both are classified as neurodevelopmental movement disorders. Tics are sudden, repetitive movements or sounds that a person feels compelled to make. When they last more than a year and involve both motor and vocal components, we call it Tourette's Syndrome.

The causes? Once again: *"unknown,"* they say. But what do scientists admit behind closed doors?

"Tics are often preceded by neuroinflammatory triggers, autoimmune reactivity, or environmental exposures in genetically susceptible individuals."
– Journal of Neuroinflammation

Sound familiar?

Let's start with the official documents:

- The MMR vaccine package insert (Merck) lists "tics" as a reported adverse event.
- The DTaP insert (Sanofi) includes "encephalopathy, seizures, and movement disorders."
- Even the HPV vaccine inserts (Gardasil) include reports of "motor tics" and "neurological complications."

So yes, they're listed. In plain sight.

And in 2010, the CDC itself published a study linking thimerosal exposure to an increased risk of tics. The study, in *Pediatric Neurology*, found:

> *"Thimerosal exposure in early infancy was significantly associated with the development of tics."*[48]

So, they knew.

And yet... the standard response is still: "No evidence of harm."

What About Vaccine Court?

Yes, there have been tic-related and Tourette's-like symptoms adjudicated in vaccine court, especially when accompanied by seizures, encephalopathy, or autism diagnoses. Here's how it typically plays out:

- A child receives a routine vaccine (often MMR, DTaP, or a combo).
- Within days or weeks, the child begins to develop involuntary movements, eye-blinking, vocal outbursts, or repetitive tics.
- Some regress cognitively. Others are diagnosed with PANDAS (pediatric autoimmune neuropsychiatric disorders associated with streptococcal infections)—a cousin to vaccine-triggered immune activation.
- The family files a claim with the National Vaccine Injury Compensation Program.
- In some cases, they are awarded compensation, not because Tourette's is "officially" recognized, but because the resulting brain injury is.

In other words, if the tic disorder is part of a larger post-vaccine encephalopathy, *compensation happens quietly.*

So What's the Mechanism? We already know:

- Aluminum adjuvants stimulate the immune system to attack foreign proteins—but sometimes they cross the blood-brain barrier and trigger chronic neuroinflammation.
- Thimerosal is neurotoxic and known to interfere with dopaminergic function, which is key in tic and Tourette's disorders.
- Polysorbate 80 helps other chemicals penetrate the brain—a chemical enabler.
- And once again: developing brains are the most vulnerable to this kind of immune provocation.

Is every case of Tourette's caused by vaccines? Of course not. But are vaccines an overlooked environmental trigger for a growing number of children developing tics and movement disorders after injections?

Let's just say: when it's listed in the insert, appears in peer-reviewed studies, and gets paid out in vaccine court... it's no longer a conspiracy—it's documented.

So we began this chapter with a simple, undeniable fact: the vaccine schedule has exploded.

In the 1950s, a child received 4 or 5 shots by age 6. Today, they'll receive over 70 doses before adulthood, many in the first year of life, when their brain, immune system, and detox pathways are still under construction.

And as that number climbed, so did the charts for chronic illness.

It's no longer "rare" to know a child with autism. Or a teen with seizures. Or a classmate with life-threatening food allergies, Tourette's, or a diagnosis like ADHD, MS, or PANDAS. And we're now told that this is just the "new normal". But we're not buying it.

We've walked through a long and disturbing list of conditions. From Guillain-Barré Syndrome, Encephalitis, Alzheimer's, and Autism, to Multiple Sclerosis, Parkinson's Disease, Allergies, Tics, Tourette's, and Seizures. And I've shown how they're all neurological, inflammatory, or autoimmune in nature. Which also happens to be exactly what vaccine ingredients can trigger.

We're talking about mercury, aluminum, formaldehyde, polysorbate 80, phenol, animal proteins, human DNA fragments, and other substances that can inflame the brain, cross the blood-brain barrier, scramble the immune system, and sometimes cause permanent damage.

Not "maybe." Not "conspiracy." These are documented facts, many admitted in vaccine package inserts, and some even compensated in vaccine court.

Besides, how can we calculate a meaningful "risk vs. benefit" when we're told the risks don't exist? When parents report seizures or regression within hours of shots and are told it's "just a coincidence"? When science admits environmental triggers can spark diseases like Parkinson's and MS, yet refuses to investigate vaccines as one of those triggers?

That's not medicine. That's marketing.

And the official line remains: "The benefits outweigh the risks." And you'll hear it over, and over, and over again ad nauseam.

But now you know. Now you can make an educated decision on whether you feel the benefits actually do outweigh the risks, or if the risks outweigh any benefits.

This isn't anti-science. This is pro-truth, pro-accountability, and pro-parental sovereignty. And I believe that every family deserves to make truly informed decisions, based on complete data, not pharmaceutical spin.

Because if the risks are real, and they are, then the choice to vaccinate should be just that: a choice. Not a mandate. Not a guilt trip. Not a threat to your job, education, or access to public life.

Now that we've opened the door to the real risks, it's time to take a closer look at an even more serious fact. Brace yourself, because Truth #5 is BIG.

Chapter Sources

1. Wakefield, A. J., et al. (1998). Ileal-lymphoid-nodular hyperplasia, non-specific colitis, and pervasive developmental disorder in children. *The Lancet*. [Retracted]
2. Hooker, B. S. (2014). Measles-mumps-rubella vaccination timing and autism among young African American boys: A reanalysis of CDC data. *Translational Neurodegeneration*, 3(1), 16.
3. Maenner, M. J., et al. (2023). Prevalence and characteristics of autism spectrum disorder among children aged 8 years — Autism and Developmental Disabilities Monitoring Network. *MMWR*, 72(2), 1–10.
4. Tomljenovic, L., & Shaw, C. A. (2011). *Do aluminum vaccine adjuvants contribute to the rising prevalence of autism?*. Journal of Inorganic Biochemistry, 105(11), 1489–1499.
5. Tomljenovic, L., & Shaw, C. A. (2012). *Mechanisms of aluminum adjuvant toxicity and autoimmunity in pediatric populations*. Lupus, 21(2), 223–230.
6. DeLong, G. (2011). *A positive association found between autism prevalence and childhood vaccination uptake across the U.S. population*. Journal of Toxicology and Environmental Health, Part A, 74(14), 903–916.
7. Shoenfeld, Y., & Agmon-Levin, N. (2011). 'ASIA'—Autoimmune/inflammatory syndrome induced by adjuvants. Journal of Autoimmunity, 36(1), 4–8.
8. Tomljenovic, L., & Shaw, C. A. (2011). Mechanisms of aluminum adjuvant toxicity and autoimmunity in pediatric populations. Lupus, 21(2), 223–230.

9. Soriano, A., & Shoenfeld, Y. (2015). Predicting post-vaccination autoimmunity: Who might be at risk?. Pharmacological Research, 92, 18–22.
10. Hayter, S. M., & Cook, M. C. (2012). Updated assessment of the prevalence, spectrum and case definition of autoimmune disease. Autoimmunity Reviews, 11(10), 754–765.
11. Lerner, G. E., Jeremias, J., & Matthias, T. (2015). The World Incidence and Prevalence of Autoimmune Diseases is Increasing. International Journal of Celiac Disease, 3(4), 151–155.
12. Exley, C. (2013). Human exposure to aluminium. *Environmental Science: Processes & Impacts*, 15(10), 1807–1816.
13. Tomljenovic, L., & Shaw, C. A. (2011). Aluminum vaccine adjuvants: Are they safe? *Current Medicinal Chemistry*, 18(17), 2630–2637.
14. Shaw, C. A., & Tomljenovic, L. (2013). Administration of aluminum to neonatal mice in vaccine-relevant amounts is associated with adverse long-term neurological outcomes. *Journal of Inorganic Biochemistry*, 128, 237–244.
15. Gherardi, R. K., Aouizerate, J., Cadusseau, J., Yara, S., Authier, F. J., & Eidi, H. (2015). Biopersistence and brain translocation of aluminum adjuvants of vaccines. *Frontiers in Neurology*, 6, 4.
16. Mold, M., Umar, D., King, A., & Exley, C. (2018). Aluminum in brain tissue in autism. *Journal of Trace Elements in Medicine and Biology*, 46, 76–82.
17. Flarend, R. E., Hem, S. L., White, J. L., Elmore, D., Suckow, M. A., Rudy, A. C., & Dandashli, F. (1997). In vivo absorption of aluminum-containing vaccine adjuvants using 26Al. Vaccine, 15(12-13), 1314–1318.

18. National Institute on Aging. (2023, May 9). Parkinson's disease: Causes, symptoms, and treatments. U.S. Department of Health & Human Services, National Institutes of Health.
19. Parkinson's Foundation. (2024). *Statistics*.
20. Bower, J. H., Maraganore, D. M., McDonnell, S. K., & Rocca, W. A. (1999). *Incidence and distribution of parkinsonism in Olmsted County, Minnesota, 1976–1990. Neurology, 52*(6), 1214–1220.
21. Dorsey, E. R., Sherer, T., Okun, M. S., & Bloem, B. R. (2018). *The rise of Parkinson's disease and its impact on society. The Lancet Neurology, 17*(11), 939–953.
22. National Multiple Sclerosis Society. (2024). *MS Prevalence*.
23. National Institutes of Health. (2022). *Multiple Sclerosis: Hope through research*. National Institute of Neurological Disorders and Stroke.
24. Petrik, M. S., Wong, M. C., Tabata, R. C., Garry, R. F., & Shaw, C. A. (2007). *Aluminum adjuvant linked to motor neuron death in mice. Neuromolecular Medicine, 9*(1), 83–100.
25. Seneff, S., Davidson, R. M., & Lauritzen, A. (2012). *Empirical data confirm autism symptoms related to aluminum and acetaminophen exposure. Entropy, 14*(11), 2227–2253.
26. WHO Multiple Sclerosis Fact Sheet (2023). *Epidemiology of MS*. World Health Organization.
27. Zhou, Y., Xu, H., Xu, W., Wang, B., Wu, Y., & Jiang, Y. (2011). *Effects of phenol on the central nervous system: Mechanisms and implications*. Journal of Hazardous Materials, 186(2–3), 1873–1880.
28. Centers for Disease Control and Prevention. (2023). *Immunization schedules*. U.S. Department of Health and Human Services.
29. Bernstein, I. L., Li, J. T., Bernstein, D. I., Hamilton, R., Spector, S. L., Tan, R., ... & Nicklas, R. A. (2003). *Allergy diagnostic testing:*

An updated practice parameter. *Annals of Allergy, Asthma & Immunology, 90*(6), 1–90.
30. Bunyavanich, S., & Schadt, E. E. (2015). Systems biology of allergy and asthma: Finding the signals amidst the noise. Nature Immunology, 16(7), 705–711.
31. Decker, M. D., Edwards, K. M., & Bogaerts, H. H. (2009). *Combination vaccines: Pros and cons. Pediatric Drugs, 11*(1), 11–23.
32. FARE (Food Allergy Research & Education). (2024). *Facts and statistics.*
33. Kumar, D., & Guyer, B. (1995). Food proteins used in vaccine manufacture may be hidden in the final product: A possible cause of food allergy. Clinical & Experimental Allergy, 25(3), 343–345.
34. Latha, M. S., & Sripathi, K. (2017). *Peanut oil and its possible role in anaphylaxis. Indian Journal of Allergy, Asthma and Immunology, 31*(1), 37–40.
35. National Institute of Allergy and Infectious Diseases. (2022). *Guidelines for the diagnosis and management of food allergy.*
36. Sicherer, S. H., & Sampson, H. A. (2018). Food allergy: A review and update on epidemiology, pathogenesis, diagnosis, prevention, and management. Journal of Allergy and Clinical Immunology, 141(1), 41–58.
37. Vinuya, R. Z., & De la Cruz, R. G. (2002). Vaccination and allergy: Is there a link? Journal of Allergy and Clinical Immunology, 110(5), 805–806.
38. Agency for Toxic Substances and Disease Registry. (1999). *Toxicological profile for mercury.* U.S. Department of Health and Human Services.

39. Agency for Toxic Substances and Disease Registry. (2008). *Toxicological profile for aluminum*. U.S. Department of Health and Human Services.
40. Davidson, A. M., Berkovic, S. F., & Scheffer, I. E. (2007). Vaccination and epilepsy: Current evidence and clinical practice. *Neurology, 68*(16), 1374–1381.
41. Geier, D. A., & Geier, M. R. (2004). Neurodevelopmental disorders following thimerosal-containing childhood immunizations: A follow-up analysis. International Journal of Toxicology, 23(6), 369–376.
42. Institute of Medicine. (2012). *Adverse effects of vaccines: Evidence and causality*. National Academies Press.
43. Jin, R., & Bo, Y. (2020). Association of vaccination with febrile seizures in children: A systematic review and meta-analysis. Scientific Reports, 10, 2113.
44. National Institute of Neurological Disorders and Stroke. (2023). *Seizures and epilepsy: Hope through research*.
45. Poling, J. S., Frye, R. E., Shoffner, J., & Zimmerman, A. W. (2006). Developmental regression and mitochondrial dysfunction in a child with autism. Journal of Child Neurology, 21(2), 170–172.
46. U.S. Health Resources and Services Administration. (2023). *Vaccine Injury Table*. National Vaccine Injury Compensation Program.
47. Barile, J. P., Kuper, D. J., Liu, G., Wong, H., & Thompson, W. W. (2012). Thimerosal exposure in early life and neuropsychological outcomes 7–10 years later. Pediatrics, 130(2), e349–e366.
48. Centers for Disease Control and Prevention. (2010). Update: Vaccine side effects, adverse reactions, contraindications, and precautions. In Epidemiology and Prevention of Vaccine-Preventable Diseases (12th ed.).

49. Geier, D. A., Hooker, B. S., Kern, J. K., & Geier, M. R. (2015). A two-phase study evaluating the relationship between Thimerosal-containing vaccine administration and the risk for an autism spectrum disorder diagnosis in the United States. Translational Neurodegeneration, 4(1), 6.
50. Merck & Co., Inc. (2023). *MMR II [Package Insert]*.
51. Sanofi Pasteur. (2023). *Daptacel (DTaP) [Package Insert]*.
52. U.S. Department of Health and Human Services. (2023). *Vaccine Injury Compensation Program: Injury Table*.
53. U.S. Court of Federal Claims. (2007). Poling v. Secretary of Health and Human Services, Case No. 02-1466V.
54. Williams, B. L., Hornig, M., Buie, T., Bauman, M. L., Cho Paik, M., Wick, I., ... & Lipkin, W. I. (2011). Impaired carbohydrate digestion and transport and mucosal dysbiosis in the intestines of children with autism and gastrointestinal disturbances. PLoS ONE, 6(12), e24585.
55. Haley, B. E. (2005). Mercury toxicity: Genetic susceptibility and synergistic effects. *Medical Veritas*, 2, 535–542.
56. Exley, C., Mold, M. J., et al. (2018). Aluminium in brain tissue in familial Alzheimer's disease. Frontiers in Neurology, 9, 666.

Chapter 8: Truth #5 - Vaccines Can—and Do—Cause Serious Harm

(You won't hear this in a pediatrician's waiting room, but it's true.)

"Vaccines injure and kill?!"

That's a bold statement, right? Maybe even the tipping point between fact and conspiracy theory?

I get it. I really do. I wish it weren't true.

I love science. I believe in innovation. I believe in using technology and knowledge to move humanity forward. So yes, I wish vaccines were safe! I wish they didn't harm or kill. I wish this chapter didn't need to be written. I wish this *book* didn't need to be written.

But we don't live in a world of wishes.

We live in a world where science can be twisted, technology can be exploited, and noble ideas, like protecting children, can be hijacked by corporations chasing profit.

We live in a world where truth is buried under lobbying, data is filtered through agendas, and the public is sold half-truths wrapped in marketing.

And in that world, we inject toxic substances into babies... while telling their parents it's for their own good.

Not for the health of the children, but for the health of the bottom line. Not for the people, but for the profit of the shareholders.

This chapter doesn't exist because I want it to.

It exists because the truth does.

Let's get something straight right now:

If vaccines were truly "safe and effective," there would be no need for a federal Vaccine Injury Compensation Program.

There would be no government-funded payout system for people who were maimed, paralyzed, or killed.

There would be no need to protect vaccine manufacturers from lawsuits.

And there certainly wouldn't be over $5 billion paid (and counting) to victims and their families—quietly, behind closed doors.

But here we are.

The phrase "vaccines save lives" has been etched into the public consciousness like gospel. It's catchy, it's comforting, and it shuts down the conversation before it ever begins. But peel back that polished slogan and something far more unsettling comes into view: vaccines also take lives. They injure. They disable. They leave devastation in their wake—and it's not just "one in a million."

Yet somehow, we've learned to excuse it. We've learned to rationalize it. It's as if society has developed a kind of psychological bond with its pharmaceutical captors—a collective Stockholm Syndrome where loyalty to the very industry profiting from our dependency feels like virtue. We defend it. We even fight for it. All while ignoring the harm that stares us in the face.

The U.S. government knows this. In fact, they codified it into law.

In 1986, Congress passed a bill that most people have never even heard of: the *National Childhood Vaccine Injury Act*. It quietly stripped families of the right to sue vaccine makers directly. It handed *legal immunity* to pharmaceutical companies. And in return? The government set up a "no-fault" system, meaning if your child dies after a shot, you can't sue the company

> "If vaccines were perfectly safe, we wouldn't need a federal compensation program for the people they injure and kill."

who made it, but you might be allowed to petition a federal board to hear your case.

That's not accountability. That's a cover-up with a payout.

So the next time someone says, "But vaccines are safe," you might ask: "If that's true… why does an entire government program exist to handle all the people they've harmed?"

In this chapter, we're going to shine a bright light on the dark reality that most people have never been told: *the injury is real, the deaths are real, and the government knows it.*

We'll walk through the laws that protect the industry, the systems that track the injuries, and the compensation program that proves this isn't theory, it's fact.

Because if even one child is injured or killed by a product the government says is required... shouldn't we all be asking: *where's the accountability?*

The Deal That Changed Everything: The True Story Behind the National Childhood Vaccine Injury Act of 1986

You know something's up when Big Pharma tells the government: "We can't keep making vaccines unless you protect us from lawsuits."

That's exactly what happened in the early 1980s, and it led to one of the most consequential, under-the-radar federal laws of the 20th century: the *National Childhood Vaccine Injury Act of 1986.*

This was the law that *quietly rewrote the rules.* It created the illusion of accountability through a government-run injury compensation program... *while giving pharmaceutical companies immunity from being sued in regular court.* And most people don't even know it exists.

The Backstory: When Parents Started Fighting Back

Let's rewind to the 1970s and early 1980s. The whole situation started boiling over around one particular vaccine: the DPT (Diphtheria, Pertussis, Tetanus) shot. Parents all over the country were reporting horrifying reactions, seizures, brain damage, and deaths, especially after the whole-cell pertussis component. Lawsuits started stacking up.

By the early '80s, vaccine injury lawsuits were hitting the manufacturers hard! Not hundreds, but thousands of claims. One of the most high-profile cases was Michael B. v. American Cyanamid in 1984, where a jury awarded over $1 million (equivalent to $3.1 million today) to the parents of a child left with severe brain damage after a DPT shot.

Suddenly, vaccine makers saw the writing on the wall. Companies like Wyeth, Connaught, and Lederle Labs started saying they might just pull out of the vaccine business altogether unless they were protected from legal liability. And the U.S. government panicked.

Enter: the American Academy of Pediatrics (AAP), the American Medical Association (AMA), and the Centers for Disease Control and Prevention (CDC). These organizations weren't neutral. They lobbied heavily, not on behalf of injured children, but to make sure vaccines stayed on the market, no matter the cost.

- The AAP, in 1984, sent a letter to Congress urging them to shield manufacturers from liability, warning that pediatricians couldn't keep vaccinating children if there were no vaccines available.[1]
- The AMA also endorsed legal immunity for manufacturers, claiming public health would be at risk if production halted.[2]
- And the CDC, while not directly writing policy, applied pressure by forecasting massive public health fallout if vaccines became unavailable due to lawsuits.[3,4]

Pharmaceutical companies, meanwhile, were flexing their muscles behind the scenes, threatening to stop making vaccines altogether unless they were protected from lawsuits. Congress caved.

The Timeline: How the 1986 Act Took Shape

- 1982: NBC airs *DPT: Vaccine Roulette*, a groundbreaking documentary exposing vaccine injuries and lawsuits. Public outrage begins to grow.
- 1984–1985: Lawsuit pressure peaks. Wyeth and Lederle threaten to leave the vaccine market.
- 1985: The first versions of the National Vaccine Injury Compensation legislation are introduced in Congress.

- November 14, 1986: Congress passes Public Law 99-660, including Title XXI—The National Childhood Vaccine Injury Act of 1986.
- November 14, 1986: President Ronald Reagan signs it into law, reluctantly, after voicing concerns about removing accountability from vaccine makers.[7]
- October 1988: The Vaccine Injury Compensation Program (VICP) officially begins processing claims.

And just like that, vaccine manufacturers were no longer liable for injuries caused by vaccines listed on the childhood schedule.

The Quiet Trade-Off: Your Child vs. Corporate Immunity

In theory, the law created a government-run "no-fault" system to fairly compensate families of injured children. But in practice?

- You can't sue the manufacturer.
- You can't sue your doctor.
- You can only petition a panel of government-appointed special masters, and only under very strict circumstances.
- Less than 1% of adverse reactions are ever even reported (via VAERS).[8,9,10]
- And yet, over $5 billion in compensation has already been paid out.[6]

Let that sink in: the system is so under-reported, so tightly regulated, and so difficult to win. Yet still, billions have been paid for *injuries and deaths* the government acknowledges were caused by vaccines.

So next time someone says vaccine injury is "rare," you might ask: *"If that's true, why did Congress have to protect the manufacturers from being sued?"*

This wasn't about health. This was about liability, reputation, and money. And the truth is, vaccine manufacturers didn't earn the public's trust. They lobbied Congress to buy it.

Now, let's do the math. Nothing too crazy, just enough to make your blood boil.

As of now, the National Vaccine Injury Compensation Program has quietly paid out over $5 billion to families whose loved ones were injured or killed by vaccines.

That's **five. billion. dollars.** From a government fund. For injuries that, we're told, are "rare."

So rare, apparently, that they needed to create a whole separate court system just to deal with them.

But here's where it gets wild.

As I previously stated, according to a federal study funded by the Department of Health and Human Services (yes, the government itself), *fewer than 1% of vaccine injuries are ever even reported to VAERS* (the Vaccine Adverse Event Reporting System).

Let that settle for a second.

If $5 billion has been paid out based on fewer than 1% of cases... what would that number look like if all injuries were actually reported?

Well, if 1% = $5 billion...
then 100% = $500 billion.
That's half a trillion dollars! (And remember: that's just what's been compensated so far, under a system designed to be nearly impossible to win.)

So when someone shrugs and says, "Well, every medical procedure has risks," you might want to reply with: *"Sure, but how many medical procedures would bankrupt the country if we actually counted all the people they hurt?"*

> If $5 billion has been paid out based on fewer than 1% of cases... what would that number look like if all injuries were actually reported?
>
> Well, if 1% = $5 billion...
> then 100% = $500 billion
>
> Vaccines don't just come with risk.
>
> **They come with a $500 billion unspoken price tag— and we've only been footing 1% of the bill.**

Vaccines don't just come with risk. They come with a $500 billion unspoken price tag—and we've only been footing 1% of the bill.

Let's stop pretending. If vaccines were truly "safe and effective" in the absolute, unquestionable way we've been told, then why does the U.S. government have an entire network of systems built around tracking, compensating, and quietly managing the harm they cause?

Seriously! Step back and just look at this logically.

We're told, *"Severe reactions are rare,"* but the federal government felt the need to create all of this:

- The **National Childhood Vaccine Injury Act of 1986**, which removed all liability from vaccine manufacturers and acknowledged, in black-and-white law, that injuries and death do happen.
- The **Vaccine Adverse Event Reporting System (VAERS)**, a government-run database to collect reports of hospitalizations, seizures, paralysis, and deaths following vaccination. If vaccines were harmless, what exactly are we tracking?
- The **Vaccine Injury Compensation Program (VICP)**, a shadow court where you can plead your case, but only if you've been injured by a vaccine the government recommends. You can't sue the manufacturer. You can't sue your doctor. You sue the federal government... and hope for a payout.
- The **Vaccine Safety Datalink**, an internal database used by the CDC to monitor possible side effects, because apparently VAERS wasn't enough. (Too many "rare" reactions?)
- And the **National Vaccine Injury Compensation Fund**, a pool of tax money collected through a $0.75 excise tax on *every* vaccine dose. That's right: your child gets a shot, and you pay into a fund to pay for the people who get injured or die.

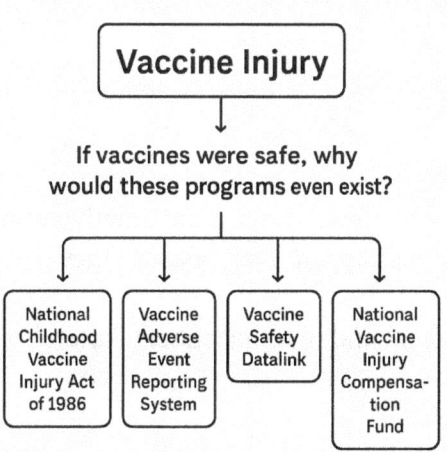

Now I ask you, if vaccines were truly as safe as the media, medical authorities, and pharmaceutical lobby want you to believe... *why would these programs even exist?*

- You don't build an entire legal infrastructure, a federal payout fund, a real-time adverse event database, and a specialized surveillance network unless you know there's a risk.
- You don't protect companies from lawsuits unless you know they could lose.
- You don't create a fund to compensate victims... unless there are victims!

So no, you don't get to say "vaccines are safe" and then turn around and defend the existence of multiple government institutions whose sole purpose is to mop up the damage.

If vaccines were safe, and if they didn't injure or kill, then none of this would be necessary.

But they're not safe. They do injure. They do kill.

And that's why these systems are quietly sitting in place, not because injuries *might* happen... but because they *do*. Every single day.

Yet the medical and pharmaceutical cartels continue to argue that point.

They say things like, *"But vaccines save far more people than they hurt."*

Really? Really?!

In the last chapter, I laid out, clearly and unapologetically, how the *risks of vaccines far outweigh any marginal benefits* they may offer.

And back in Chapter 4, we dismantled the myth of vaccine derived herd immunity. Using data, logic, and critical thinking, I showed how vaccines don't create it, they *suppress* it. They block the natural immunity process and keep the population tethered to a multi-billion dollar system built on perpetual injections and corporate dependency.

But despite all of this, the argument keeps coming: "The benefits to the many, outweigh the risks to the few."

Well, I argue this:

Every number has a name. Every one of the "few" is someone's child.

So, let's talk numbers. Because while the government doesn't exactly put this on a billboard, it's all publicly available if you know where to look.

Since the Vaccine Injury Compensation Program (VICP) started in 1988, over $5.2 billion has been paid out to people who were injured or killed by vaccines. That's not opinion, that's from the *U.S. Health Resources & Services Administration* (HRSA).

So how many people does that actually represent?

As of mid-2024, *more than 10,000 individuals* have been officially compensated for vaccine injuries or deaths. That's ten thousand lives! Ten thousand families who went through the system and won their case (or settled before it finished).

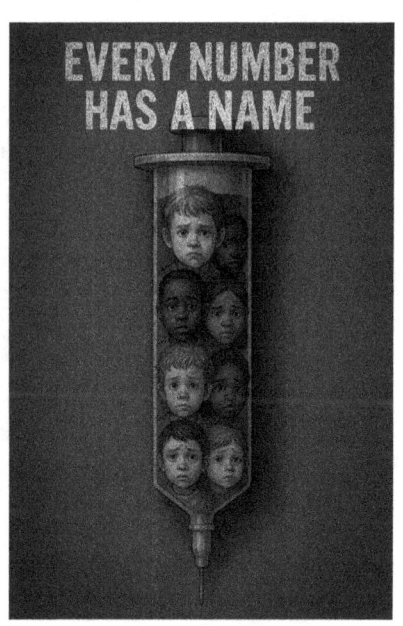

Now here's the kicker: those are just the people who *made it through the process!*

The system is tough to navigate. You can't sue in regular court. You file a claim with the federal government, and if you're lucky, they'll agree that a vaccine hurt you or your child.

And what about everyone else?

Well, according to a federal study funded by the HHS (not some fringe group), less than 1% of vaccine injuries are ever even reported to VAERS—the system that feeds into the Vaccine Injury Compensation Program (VICP).

So if 10,000 people were compensated, and that's based on less than 1% of actual injuries being reported... you do the math.

We're looking at *hundreds of thousands,* possibly *millions*, of vaccine injuries and deaths. But sure... tell me again how "rare" it is.

So here we are.

Not speculating. Not wondering. Not asking *if* vaccines injure and kill.

We've seen the data. We've walked through the logic. We've followed the paper trail. And the conclusion is crystal clear: Vaccines do injure. Vaccines do kill.

Not "rarely."

They do.

And the numbers? They're not small.

They're not some abstract data point in a distant database. They're *staggeringly immense.* So immense, in fact, it's hard to even grasp.

But let's try.

Let's take off the white coats, shut down the spreadsheets, and talk human to human.

Over $5 billion has already been paid out in compensation. And that's with a system that, by its own admission, captures less than 1% of adverse events. So again, multiply that.

Now imagine, buried in that flood of cases… is *your* child. *Your* niece. *Your* grandson.

Maybe that's why you picked up this book in the first place—because you *know* something happened.

You *know* your child changed after that shot.

And you were told, "It's just coincidence."

But you didn't buy it.

Because every number has a name.

Every statistic has (or had) a heartbeat.

What if that name… was the one you whispered into your newborn baby's ear when they were born?

You don't need to imagine this in the abstract. The odds don't live in some far-off place.

In just *one* of the neurological conditions I spoke about in this book, the odds are 1 in 36 children.

That's tens of thousands in your state. Thousands in your cities. Dozens in your school district. One or two in every classroom.

This isn't "rare."

This is personal.

This is *your neighborhood*.

This is your family.

So why, despite all of this, do the media, the government, the medical system, and pharmaceutical giants continue to pretend this risk is insignificant?

Why are these injuries treated as "acceptable losses"?

Why don't they seem to care?

Well, that's what we're going to unpack next.

Because behind every dose… every mandate… every dismissal of a parent's pain… there's something else at play:

Get ready for Truth #6 , because there is financial incentive to vaccines.

Chapter Sources

1. Colgrove, J. (2006). *State of Immunity: The Politics of Vaccination in Twentieth-Century America*. University of California Press.
2. Hinman, A. R., Orenstein, W. A., & Mortimer, E. A. (1992). *Vaccination and the law. Law, Medicine & Health Care, 20(1–2), 9–14. (2015). History of Vaccine Safety.*
3. Institute of Medicine (US) Committee on the Children's Vaccine Initiative. (1993). *The Children's Vaccine Initiative: Achieving the Vision*. National Academies Press.
4. Baker, J. P. (2008). *The vaccine compensation system. New England Journal of Medicine, 357(19), 1965–1967.*
5. Institute of Medicine. (1991). *Adverse Effects of Pertussis and Rubella Vaccines*. National Academy Press.
6. National Vaccine Injury Compensation Program (VICP). (2023). *HRSA Data & Statistics*. U.S. Department of Health and Human Services.
7. Reagan, R. (1986, November 14). *Statement on signing the National Childhood Vaccine Injury Act of 1986*. Ronald Reagan Presidential Library.
8. Lazarus, R., & Klompas, M. (2010). Electronic Support for Public Health–Vaccine Adverse Event Reporting System (ESP:VAERS) Final Report. Harvard Pilgrim Health Care, Inc., for the U.S. Department of Health and Human Services (HHS).
9. Rosenthal, S., Chen, R. T. (1995). The reporting sensitivities of two passive surveillance systems for vaccine adverse events. American Journal of Public Health, 85(12), 1706–1709.

10. Shimabukuro, T. T., Nguyen, M., Martin, D., & DeStefano, F. (2015). Safety monitoring in the Vaccine Adverse Event Reporting System (VAERS). Vaccine, 33(36), 4398–4405.

Chapter 9: Truth #6 - There's Big Money Behind Every Shot

(When billions are on the line, safety becomes negotiable.)

"The hypocrisy of some is that we like to think of ourselves as sophisticated and evolved, but we're still also driven by primal urges like greed and power"

—Michael Leunig

Let's not pretend this is about your child's health anymore.

Let's stop pretending this is some noble crusade by modern medicine to protect humanity from invisible germs. Because if it were truly about health, if it were really about preventing harm, you wouldn't need to pay people to inject poison into children. You wouldn't need financial bribes to prop up a system built on half-truths and silenced science. And yet, that's exactly where we are.

Vaccines are not just a product. They're not even just a medical intervention. They are a financial empire. A booming, high-margin, high-growth cash machine for some of the most powerful industries on Earth. The pharmaceutical industry has built a product line that is not only immune from liability thanks to the National Childhood Vaccine Injury Act of 1986, but also *guaranteed* by government purchase and pushed through every public health agency, school system, and media outlet in the country.

It's the perfect business model. No refunds. No lawsuits. No responsibility. Just repeat customers with guaranteed demand, starting on day one of life.

So how big is this business, exactly?

In 1980, the global vaccine market was worth less than a billion dollars.[1] Chump change compared to what it's become. Today, estimates place the vaccine industry's value at over $70 billion annually[2], and it's projected to hit $125 billion within the next few years[3]. Pfizer alone brought in $37.8 billion in 2022 from its COVID-19 vaccine[4,5], more than double what it earned from all of its vaccine products combined in 2019. Moderna made $18.4 billion in a single year off one vaccine[6]. These aren't figures from a public health initiative. These are revenue reports from a pharmaceutical gold rush.

And when that kind of money is on the table, people don't play fair. They don't tell the truth. They sell stories. They buy silence. And they legislate profits.

Let's talk about legislation. You probably assume your elected officials are working for you. That they weigh the science, look at the data, and make informed decisions in the interest of public safety. You'd be wrong. Because in Washington, loyalty is rented by the highest bidder. And guess who's doing the bidding?

In 2022 alone, the pharmaceutical industry spent over $372 million on lobbying in the United States[7]... more than any other industry by a landslide. That's over a million dollars a day to influence lawmakers, shape public health policy, and keep the vaccine train rolling.

Members of Congress don't just vote on health laws. They *profit* from them. They own stock in the very companies they're supposed to regulate.[8,9,10,11,12] They sit on committees that determine vaccine mandates while receiving campaign contributions from the manufacturers who stand to benefit. And nobody calls it a conflict of interest. Because that's not what they call it in D.C.... they call it business as usual.

It's no coincidence that vaccine mandates get tighter, the schedule gets longer, and resistance gets labeled as extremism. This is not about science. It's about sales.

And it doesn't stop at Congress.

Let's talk about doctors. You probably think your pediatrician makes vaccine recommendations because they believe it's the best choice for your child. Maybe that's true. But what's also true is that there's money in it. Not just reimbursement for administering the shot, but *bonuses*! Cold, hard, incentive-driven bonuses paid by insurance companies to physicians for meeting vaccine quotas.

Take Blue Cross Blue Shield of Michigan, for example. In 2016, a spokesperson admitted that pediatricians could receive bonuses ranging anywhere from $400 to $9,600 for meeting childhood vaccination targets. One specific target? Ensuring that at least 63% of their pediatric patients were fully vaccinated by age 2. If they hit that mark, they got paid.[13]

Let me say that again. Doctors were financially rewarded. Not for better outcomes, not for healthier kids, but for compliance with the vaccine schedule. And what was on that schedule? Hepatitis B on the first day of life, rotavirus, polio, MMR, DTaP, varicella, pneumococcal—dozens of doses by age two. And if you refused? If you delayed? That was one less point for your pediatrician's bonus calculation.

Do other insurers do this? Absolutely. A review of Medicaid Managed Care incentive programs shows that multiple states, including New York, California, and Illinois, offer financial rewards tied directly to childhood vaccine coverage rates.[14,15,16,17] The amounts vary. The strings are always the same. It's about hitting numbers, not individualizing care. It's about keeping score with syringes.

According to a 2021 review by the Office of Inspector General (OIG), "Many Medicaid Managed Care Organizations tie provider bonus payments to vaccine adherence measures."[18] These are the very organizations that administer care to millions of low-income children across the country. Meaning the kids with the least say in their care are being used as metrics in a spreadsheet, with doctors pocketing bonuses for compliance.

And the kicker? These payments aren't even secret. They're just never disclosed to the parents. The same people who are told, "This is safe, this is necessary, this is for your child's protection," are never told, "Oh, and your doctor gets a cash bonus if you say yes."

The system is so saturated with financial incentives that questioning it becomes dangerous—not just to the profit margins, but to the power structures that rely on it. That's why skeptics are demonized. That's why scientific dissenters are censored. That's why whistleblowers are silenced and data is buried.

The vaccine program isn't failing. It's thriving.

It's just not thriving for you.

It's thriving for pharmaceutical executives who sit on their yachts while vaccine-injured children sit in therapy sessions their parents can barely afford. It's thriving for insurance companies who run spreadsheets instead of health plans. It's thriving for lawmakers who count contributions, not casualties.

This isn't conspiracy. This is capitalism on steroids, protected by regulation, fueled by taxpayer dollars, and hidden behind a wall of "safe and effective" slogans. They tell you it's about public health. But follow the money and you'll find it's really about private wealth.

So the next time someone says, "Vaccines are safe," ask them who's getting paid to say it.

The next time a doctor urges another injection, ask them if they're getting a bonus check for it.

The next time a politician pushes a mandate, ask them what stock options they're holding.

And the next time you hear that questioning vaccines is dangerous, remember: the real danger lies in not questioning at all.

Now, let's peel back a few more layers.

You've probably heard of "Operation Warp Speed." Sounds heroic, doesn't it? Like a superhero sprinting toward a burning building to save the world. Except this was no act of bravery. This was $30 billion in corporate handouts[19,20] dressed up as a rescue mission. Under Warp Speed, companies like Pfizer and Moderna got billions in government funding. Not to research vaccines, not to run long-term safety trials, but to manufacture millions of doses before they even finished collecting proper data.

Again, that's not science, that's speculation backed by your tax dollars.

And guess who made off like bandits? Pfizer's CEO, for example, cashed out millions in stock the very same day his company announced positive trial data.[21] Moderna's executives? They sold off hundreds of millions in shares during the pandemic, timing sales perfectly with public announcements.[22] It's not just about saving lives. It's about maximizing return on investment. And you, your kids, your schools, and your communities, are the investment vehicle.

Even worse, the government isn't just giving money to pharma, it's guaranteeing them a market. Vaccines don't need to be good products. They don't even need to be in demand. Because government mandates and CDC recommendations ensure that millions of doses are bought, distributed, and injected—year after year—no matter what. There's no other industry like this. Imagine if Ford got paid in advance for every car, didn't have to guarantee the brakes worked, and couldn't be sued when they didn't. That's what we're dealing with here. That's what the vaccine industry has become. A government-guaranteed revenue stream—completely detached from consumer demand, product liability, or market accountability.

They don't need to advertise to convince you. The CDC does that for them. They don't need to sell to hospitals or doctors. The federal government bulk-buys doses with taxpayer money. And they don't need to worry about lawsuits when things go wrong—because they're shielded by a special legal immunity no other industry enjoys. This isn't capitalism. It's cronyism. A closed-loop cartel where the manufacturers write the playbook, the regulators enforce it, and the public foots the bill. Whether the products are safe or not doesn't even enter the equation. Whether people want them or not doesn't matter. The money keeps flowing.

So ask yourself—if the product is that good, why do they have to force it?

Why the mandates? Why the liability protection? Why the propaganda campaigns and the financial bonuses for every needle pushed into a baby's arm?

Because in a free market, bad products fail. But in the vaccine market, bad products are protected, promoted, and paid for in advance.

It's the only product where the manufacturer is immune, but you're not!

And when you look at how the system treats vaccine injuries? It gets worse. Because the government set up a separate court. One that doesn't follow the same rules, doesn't have a jury of your peers, and doesn't allow you to sue the manufacturer. You're stuck playing legal roulette with a federal tribunal that's paid out over $5 billion to date in injury claims. And that's with less than 1% of adverse events ever being reported. So if five billion dollars have already been paid out under a system where 99% of injuries go unreported, what does that really mean? That number doesn't represent the total cost of vaccine injury, it represents a tiny fraction. A sliver. A controlled leak from a dam holding back a flood of truth.

Imagine if every injured child's case actually made it through. If every parent who connected the dots and demanded justice was counted. If the system didn't intimidate doctors into silence, bury reports, or gaslight families into thinking what they saw with their own eyes *"must have been a coincidence."*

We wouldn't be talking about $5 billion. We'd be talking about hundreds of billions.

We'd be talking about one of the largest public health scandals in modern history.

But we're not. Because the "Vaccine Court" doesn't function like a real court. There's no jury. No discovery. No ability to sue the company that made the product that caused the damage. The defendants are shielded. The process is secretive. And the burden is on *you*—the parent—to prove what even the CDC admits is biologically plausible.

And still, thousands of families have been paid. Quietly. Off the books. With gag orders and settlements and decisions that never reach public consciousness.

So when they tell you vaccines are "safe and effective," you have to ask: if they're so safe, why does a shadow court even exist? And if they're so effective, why do so many families walk away with check—and broken children?

Because what they're really paying for... is silence.

This isn't theoretical. This isn't rare. This is happening to real people in real time.

And all the while, the industry keeps the narrative going by paying off the very people meant to protect you. The top 20 recipients of pharma lobbying money in Congress? They vote 100% in alignment with industry interests. The FDA and CDC? These are federal agencies that are supposed to be representing you and looking out for your best interests—because they are funded with your tax dollars. Unfortunately, their advisory panels are littered with former and future employees of vaccine manufacturers. It's a revolving door. You approve the product this year, and next year you're on the board.

What's the result? Ever-expanding vaccine schedules. In 1983, a child received 11 shots by age 5. In 2025, it's 72 doses by age 18. And guess what? More are coming. RSV, flu, COVID boosters, HPV for kids as young as 9. Why? Because every new shot is a new revenue stream. Not a new health breakthrough. Just a new billable moment.

And who's helping them push these policies at the local level? Insurance companies like Aetna and UnitedHealthcare, which quietly tie physician bonuses to vaccine rates. In California, pediatricians receive incentive payments for meeting coverage thresholds under Medi-Cal Managed Care programs.[17] In Illinois, providers are given financial boosts based on how many children receive the full CDC schedule.[18] This is widespread. And it's all cloaked under the illusion of care.

They say it's about "public health." But what they mean is: public obedience. Compliance with a system that doesn't care if your child is healthy, only if they're vaccinated.

The most sinister part? Parents aren't told about any of this. They don't know their doctor might be earning thousands for every "*yes*" they say. They don't know their politicians are funded by the very companies lobbying for mandates. They don't know that the people who determine the "standard of care" have skin in the game—and it's not your child's skin.

They don't tell you any of this. Because if they did, you might stop trusting them. And if you stop trusting them… you might stop complying. And if you stop complying? The whole tower of lies starts to crumble.

But maybe that's exactly what needs to happen.

Because we're not just talking about health. We're talking about the foundation of an industry that's become more interested in shares than science, more committed to revenue than recovery, and more loyal to stakeholders than to the people they swore to protect.

Vaccines are no longer a public service. They are a public business.

And business is booming.

Let's get specific.

In 2022, Pfizer made $37.8 billion off its COVID-19 vaccine alone. That wasn't total revenue. That was just one vaccine. That number exceeded the GDP of over 100 countries.[23,24] Moderna? $18.4 billion in 2022.[25] Remember, before COVID, most people had never heard of Moderna. It had never successfully brought a vaccine to market. But the right connections, the right narrative, and a bottomless pit of government money changed that overnight. One product. Instant empire.

Merck, known for its MMR and Gardasil vaccines, raked in nearly $9 billion in 2022 from vaccine sales.[26] Sanofi brought in over $6 billion.[27] GlaxoSmithKline, over $8 billion.[28] These aren't struggling public health departments. These are global giants built on recurring, government-supported, liability-free injections.

And each one spends millions, sometimes hundreds of millions, on marketing, lobbying, and "educational" partnerships. In fact, pharmaceutical companies as a whole spent over $6.8 billion on direct-to-consumer advertising in 2022.[29] That's what funds those constant commercials reminding you to "ask your doctor." And you *should* ask. But don't ask what the ad suggests. Ask who paid for the script.

Now, let's look at lobbying. In 2022, Big Pharma spent over $372 million on lobbying in the U.S. alone, according to OpenSecrets.[7] That money went toward influencing bills, blocking regulatory reforms, securing favorable treatment, and yes—defending vaccine mandates. You think mandates are about public health? Open your eyes. Mandates are guaranteed sales!

Let's not pretend this is about a few bad apples.

Some of the most influential figures in Congress—those who've chaired the Senate Health Committee, served on the House Energy and Commerce Committee, or led key finance and oversight panels—have direct and ongoing financial entanglements with the pharmaceutical industry.

One former Senate committee chair, for example, accepted hundreds of thousands of dollars in pharmaceutical contributions over his tenure, while holding stock in companies that stood to benefit directly from vaccine approvals. Not surprisingly, his votes aligned closely with industry interests. He wasn't just overseeing public health policy. He was positioned to *profit* from it.

Then there was the House representative who co-owned a veterinary pharmaceutical company. While serving on one of the most powerful committees shaping health legislation, he consistently voted in line with Big Pharma. When your business is drugs, and you're voting on drug policy, it's hard to pretend there's no conflict of interest. But this isn't ancient history—and it's not fringe. In 2025, during his Senate confirmation hearings for Secretary of Health and Human Services, **Robert F. Kennedy, Jr.** called this out in plain language. He pointed directly at several high-profile senators—those who've built reputations as champions of healthcare reform—yet received sizable campaign donations from the very pharmaceutical companies they claim to be regulating.

One of those senators, who routinely lectures the public on holding corporations accountable, had accepted thousands in contributions from major pharmaceutical companies throughout her career. Another, who proudly identifies as a progressive voice for justice, was funded millions by some of the same health and insurance PACs tied to the vaccine rollout and mandates.

Then came the grilling. Several senators who questioned Kennedy at that hearing had deep ties to pharma dollars themselves. One had accepted over $30,000 in a single year from PACs linked to the hospital and chemical industries. Another brought in thousands from some of the biggest pharmaceutical and insurance giants—companies like Novartis, AstraZeneca, and Bristol Myers Squibb.

And yet these individuals were allowed to sit in judgment over a man who's spent decades exposing the influence of corporate power in medicine.

Let's be clear: this isn't about isolated corruption. This is the blueprint.

When lawmakers are taking money from the very industries they're supposed to regulate—while voting on your child's health, your access to medical freedom, your bodily autonomy—you have every right to question their motives.

They tell you to "trust the science." But what they don't say is who's funding it… and who's cashing in.

The truth is, the pharmaceutical industry's grip on Congress isn't just strong—it's systemic. Dozens of lawmakers on key health committees—both Democrats and Republicans—regularly take donations from pharmaceutical manufacturers, health insurers, and hospital lobbying groups. They write the rules, accept the checks, and vote to expand the very programs that funnel taxpayer money straight into pharma's already-bloated pockets.

It's not a conspiracy theory. It's campaign finance 101.

Now back to the insurance incentives.

We've already discussed Blue Cross Blue Shield of Michigan. But they're not alone. In New York, Medicaid Managed Care organizations have performance measures tied to vaccination rates. Providers get quarterly payments based on how many of their pediatric patients are "up to date."[34] In Texas, the CHIP program includes financial rewards for hitting immunization benchmarks.[35] In Illinois, physicians in managed care plans receive incentive bonuses tied directly to compliance with the CDC childhood schedule.[36]

And here's the kicker: the CDC itself provides grant funding and infrastructure to these programs, promoting vaccine adherence as a metric of provider performance.[37] That means the same agency recommending more vaccines is helping fund the programs that reward doctors for delivering them.

It's a closed loop!

- The CDC recommends the product.
- The government buys it in bulk.
- The insurance companies reward its use.
- The pharmaceutical companies count the profits.
- And the doctors smile at their bonus checks.

You think anyone in that circle is incentivized to speak out when something goes wrong?

Let's talk about that.

What happens when a physician sees a clear vaccine injury? A febrile seizure, a regression into autism, a case of Guillain-Barré Syndrome? They're supposed to report it to VAERS, the Vaccine Adverse Event Reporting System. But here's the problem… there's no penalty for not reporting. No accountability. And every report raises the risk of being flagged as "anti-vax" by hospital administrators or state boards. In a system where silence is rewarded and questioning is punished, how much truth do you think sees the light of day?

Meanwhile, the media (funded by pharma ad dollars) keeps the public distracted with celebrity endorsements and shaming campaigns.

"Trust the science," they say. But they never mention that "the science" is being funded, written, and ghost-edited by the very companies profiting from the results.

And let's not forget the medical journals. A study published in JAMA (Journal of the American Medical Association) found that 7 out of 10 clinical trial authors had financial ties to the drug companies whose products they were evaluating.[38,39] That's not objectivity. That's marketing dressed up as medicine.

The deeper you dig, the more it stinks.

This isn't a health care system. It's a syndicate. A well-oiled machine that launders science into policy, policy into mandates, mandates into profits, and silences anyone who dares break the chain.

Doctors are paid to stay in line.

Politicians are paid to keep the laws in place.

Scientists are paid to publish the right conclusions.

And the rest of us? We're just the customers. The test subjects. The data points.

And if we dare ask questions? We're labeled conspiracy theorists. Dangerous. Unhinged. But let me ask you this: What's more unhinged? Asking why a multi-billion-dollar industry needs legal immunity and government mandates to survive? Or pretending it's normal to inject dozens of vaccines into infants before they can even speak… and rewarding doctors who do it with thousands in bonuses?

This chapter isn't about ideology. It's about economics. Vaccines are profitable. Massively profitable. And everyone at the top of the pyramid is cashing in. The only ones paying the price are the families dealing with the fallout. The ones picking up the pieces of a system designed not to care.

So yes, there is financial incentive to vaccines.

And it's the reason the system won't stop.

It's the reason your doctor doesn't ask questions.

It's the reason your lawmakers look the other way.

It's the reason your child is just one more number on a spreadsheet.

Because as long as the checks keep clearing… no one at the top has any reason to say no.

It's not speculation. It's not a theory. It's fact. Vaccines are a profit center. They generate billions, prop up institutions, fund elections, and incentivize silence. This isn't a healthcare system. It's a machine. One that needs constant fuel, in the form of compliant parents, trusting patients, and a public kept just unaware enough to not ask the right questions.

We've peeled back the layers and followed the money. What we found was predictable: when health becomes profit, ethics become optional. And that's exactly what we're up against.

You've seen the numbers. You've seen the mechanisms. You've seen how the game is rigged. Not for your benefit, but for theirs.

And yet, it gets worse.

Because even with all the money changing hands, and the power consolidating, and the injuries mounting… they still pretend this is your choice. They still put a smiling nurse in the exam room, hand you a clipboard, and act like you've just made an "informed decision."

But what if that decision was never really yours?

What if the truth was withheld from you?

What if "informed consent" was nothing more than a performance?

In the next chapter, we'll talk about exactly that.

Your doctor is required to give you this information. But what happens when they don't?

Let's find out.

Chapter Sources

1. Plotkin, S. A., Orenstein, W. A., & Offit, P. A. (2013). *Vaccines* (6th ed.). Elsevier.
2. World Health Organization. (2022). *Global Vaccine Market Report 2022*.
3. Fortune Business Insights. (2023). Vaccines Market Size, Share & Trends, 2023–2030.
4. Pfizer Inc. (2023). *Form 10-K Annual Report 2022*. U.S. Securities and Exchange Commission.
5. Pfizer Inc. (2020). *Form 10-K Annual Report 2019*. U.S. Securities and Exchange Commission.
6. Moderna Inc. (2023). *Form 10-K Annual Report 2022*. U.S. Securities and Exchange Commission.
7. OpenSecrets. (2023). Pharmaceutical / Health Products: Lobbying, 2022. Center for Responsive Politics.
8. OpenSecrets. (2022). *Stock Trading by U.S. Senators and Representatives*. Center for Responsive Politics.
9. Office of the Clerk, U.S. House of Representatives. (2023). *Periodic Transaction Reports*. U.S. House of Representatives.
10. Slodysko, B., & Fingerhut, H. (2022, December 27). *Congress members traded health and tech stocks while overseeing pandemic response*. AP News.
11. Lipton, E., & Fandos, N. (2020, March 19). *Senators Sold Stock After Coronavirus Briefings*. The New York Times.
12. Levinthal, D. (2022, February 9). Congress and conflict: Lawmakers' stock trades often match committee assignments. Business Insider.

13. Children's Health Defense. (2020, February 12). Pediatricians pushing vaccines receive bigger paychecks.
14. Medicaid and CHIP Payment and Access Commission (MACPAC). (2020). *State Medicaid managed care quality strategies: A look at immunization incentives.*
15. New York State Department of Health. (2021). Quality Incentive Program for Medicaid Managed Care Plans: Technical Specifications Manual.
16. California Department of Health Care Services (DHCS). (2022). *Managed Care Performance Measures.*
17. Illinois Department of Healthcare and Family Services. (2021). *Healthcare Quality Strategy for Managed Care Organizations.*
18. U.S. Department of Health and Human Services, Office of Inspector General. (2021, March). *Medicaid Managed Care: Incentives for Providers* (OEI-05-19-00350).
19. U.S. Government Accountability Office (GAO). (2021, January). Operation Warp Speed: Accelerated COVID-19 Vaccine Development Status and Efforts to Address Manufacturing Challenges (GAO-21-319).
20. U.S. Department of Health and Human Services (HHS). (2020, July 30). *Fact Sheet: Explaining Operation Warp Speed.*
21. Thomas, K., & Gelles, D. (2020, November 17). Pfizer's CEO sold $5.6 million in stock as company announced promising vaccine news. The New York Times.
22. Elkind, P. (2021, October 8). Moderna insiders have cashed out $3.6 billion in stock as company's value soared. STAT News.
23. Pfizer Inc. (2023, January 31). *Pfizer Reports Fourth-Quarter and Full-Year 2022 Results.*
24. World Bank. (2023). GDP (current US$).

25. Moderna, Inc. (2023, February 23). Moderna Reports Fourth Quarter and Full Year 2022 Financial Results and Provides Business Updates [Press release].
26. Merck & Co., Inc. (2023, February 2). *Merck Announces Fourth-Quarter and Full-Year 2022 Financial Results.*
27. Sanofi. (2023, February 3). *Sanofi delivers strong 2022 business EPS growth of 17.1% at CER.*
28. GSK (GlaxoSmithKline). (2023, February 1). Full year and Q4 2022 results.
29. Statista Research Department. (2023, March). Pharmaceutical industry ad spending in the United States from 2012 to 2022.
30. Federal Election Commission. (2024). Campaign Finance Individual and PAC Contributions Search: Ron Wyden, Sheldon Whitehouse, Michael Bennet.
31. Center for Responsive Politics. (2024). *Pharmaceutical/Health Products: Top Recipients.* OpenSecrets.org.
32. Lipton, E., & Sanger-Katz, M. (2021, November 13). *How the pharmaceutical industry gets its way in Washington. The New York Times.*
33. Statista Research Department. (2023, April). Top industries contributing to congressional campaigns in 2024.
34. New York State Department of Health. (2021). Quality Incentive Program for Medicaid Managed Care Plans: Technical Specifications Manual.
35. Texas Health and Human Services Commission. (2023). CHIP Performance Indicator Dashboard and Incentive Measures.
36. Illinois Department of Healthcare and Family Services. (2021). *Quality Strategy for Medicaid Managed Care.*
37. Centers for Disease Control and Prevention (CDC). (2022). Immunization and Vaccines for Children Cooperative Agreements.

38. Ross, J. S., Hill, K. P., Egilman, D. S., & Krumholz, H. M. (2008). Guest authorship and ghostwriting in publications related to rofecoxib: A case study of industry documents from litigation. Journal of the American Medical Association, 299(15), 1800–1812.
39. Bekelman, J. E., Li, Y., & Gross, C. P. (2003). Scope and impact of financial conflicts of interest in biomedical research: A systematic review. Journal of the American Medical Association, 289(4), 454–465.

Chapter 10: Truth #7 - Your Doctor Is Supposed to Tell You More—They Usually Don't

(Informed consent isn't optional. It's the law.)[1,2,3]

"Informed Consent." You've seen those two words a few times already in this book. They sound official, even noble (like the kind of thing you'd want anytime you or your child undergoes a medical procedure). And they are. Informed Consent is foundational to ethical medicine. But here's the problem: it's largely absent in how vaccines are pushed, promoted, and administered.

Let's break it down. Informed Consent isn't just about getting a patient to say "yes." It means giving a patient all the pertinent information to make an educated, voluntary choice about their care. That includes discussing the risks. The benefits. The alternatives. The option to say "no." And, when it comes to vaccinations, that includes the right to refuse… even for personal, philosophical, or conscientious reasons.

Because here's the truth: every vaccine carries the risk of injury. Some carry the risk of death. That's not opinion, that's fact—acknowledged by the very institutions that manufacture and promote vaccines. So, if a parent is going to make a truly informed choice, they have to be given that risk profile honestly and clearly. Anything less? That's coercion dressed up in a white coat.

But how can doctors inform you of risks they themselves don't know?

Let's talk about the elephant in the room: most doctors know very little about vaccines. And that's not some wild claim. That's coming from their own mouths.

I've personally interviewed MDs and pediatricians and asked them point-blank: "How much did you learn in medical school about vaccines?" The answer is always some version of: "Honestly? Nothing."

Not a class. Not a module. Not a lab. Just the broad assumption that vaccines are "safe and effective," and their job as a future doctor is to promote, schedule, and administer them. No questions asked.

Let's take a look at one of the most widely used medical textbooks in the world: *Guyton and Hall Textbook of Medical Physiology*. This thing is the bible of human physiology. Over 1,000 pages. It teaches medical students everything about how the body functions—cardiology, nephrology, neurophysiology, immunology… you name it.

And how much space is devoted to vaccination in this thousand-page tome? One paragraph.

That's it. One small paragraph in a textbook that's supposed to prepare doctors to understand and treat the human body.

There's no chapter called "Vaccination." No "Immunization 101." Just a few lines that essentially state what it is… artificial active and artificial passive immunity. Now move along.

So how can the average doctor offer informed consent when they themselves haven't been informed?

I know this firsthand. I myself have had to learn about this issue outside of formal schooling. Over the past 35+ years, I've spent literally thousands and thousands of hours researching, investigating, and studying all sides of the vaccine issue. Not just the mainstream narrative, but also the suppressed studies, the inconvenient truths, and the firsthand stories from real families. This has not been a casual interest—it's been a full-on pursuit of truth.

Meanwhile, the average medical doctor finishes their degree and immediately steps into the field to practice what they were taught. From day one, they begin repeating what they were told, without ever having truly examined it. Not because they're lazy or disinterested, but because the system is structured to reward compliance, not curiosity.

Now, before we go any further, let me be clear: **doctors are not the enemy.**

Most doctors are good people. Compassionate people. People who got into medicine because they wanted to help, to heal, to make lives better. They trust the system that trained them. They believe in the institutions that guided them. They genuinely believe they're doing what's best.

And why wouldn't they? From the moment they walk into medical school, they're told that vaccines are one of modern medicine's greatest achievements. That questioning them is not just unnecessary, it's dangerous. So it's no surprise that most doctors double down on that belief. Not out of malice. But out of *misguided trust.*

It's not their fault that they weren't taught this material. The curriculum was handed to them. The assumptions were baked in. And the pressure to conform—to follow the CDC, the AAP, and the hospital protocol—is immense. And then they enter the field.

Let me tell you something I've learned—both from research and personal experience. There are two types of pediatricians out there. Two kinds of family doctors. And it matters, deeply, which one is caring for your child.

The first type will respect your decisions. Even if your health philosophy doesn't align with theirs, they understand that their job is to gather data about your child's health, provide you with their expert opinion, and then respect your decision. These doctors operate with humility. They offer guidance, not ultimatums. They understand their role is advisory, not authoritarian. These are the good ones—the ones worth keeping.

Then there's the second kind. The ones who don't respect your philosophy. Who treat your questions like insubordination. These are the doctors who say, "Follow my orders or find another doctor." They see themselves as the final authority—above reproach, above inquiry, and above accountability. They live in a self-absorbed world where dissent is seen as defiance.

These are the doctors who will expel you from their practice if you don't vaccinate on command. But here's the thing: if that happens to you, *consider it a blessing*. You've just been given the clearest red flag possible. *That's not your doctor!* That's not your child's advocate. That's someone who's in it for themselves. Someone who cannot be trusted to put your child's best interest above their own ego.

Find the first kind. The ones who will share what they know, and listen when you share what you've learned. The ones who will partner with you, not parent you.

Because here's something the American Medical Association (AMA) has made abundantly clear: physicians are *not* ethically allowed to refuse care to a patient simply because that person is unvaccinated or chooses not to vaccinate. The AMA Code of Ethics—Opinion 8.3 and 1.1.2—states that physicians have a duty to treat even in the face of risk, and that turning a patient away based on their vaccination status is discriminatory.[4,5]

So if your pediatrician ever refuses to see your child because they're unvaccinated, they're *violating the very ethical standards of their profession.*

Is that really someone you want making medical decisions for your child?

I've seen this dynamic unfold in real time. I've gone with parents to "well-child" visits where they knew vaccines would come up—and not just casually, but with pressure. Why, because the parents unfortunately chose the second type of doctor.

I've sat in those exam rooms and watched what happens when you ask questions—real questions.

It always starts out friendly enough. "We're due for some shots today," the doctor says cheerfully. But once you start asking questions—the deep, important questions—the temperature in the room drops fast.

Ask them why they follow the CDC schedule. They'll say, "Because vaccines save lives."

Ask them if they know what's actually in the vaccine. Cue the stammering, or worse, the dismissive smile.

Ask about polysorbate 80, phenol, aluminum adjuvants, or fetal cell lines. They'll either stare at you blankly or pull out the CDC website.

Ask them about informed consent and they'll suddenly get serious—cold, even—and then ask a nurse to retrieve the vaccine package inserts. (That's the giant foldout sheet printed in microscopic font, that looks like a road map and reads like a legal waiver.) They hand it to you, not out of a sense of duty, but because they feel legally cornered.

Ask them if they've ever read a full vaccine package insert. Most will admit they haven't. And those who have? They're only handing them to you because you requested them. That's "informed consent," modern pediatrics style.

Ask what the ingredients mean, or whether they're safe, and out comes the mantra: "The benefits outweigh the risks."

Ask about the risk of your child contracting polio from the polio vaccine itself, and they'll deny it. When you cite the CDC's own data, they'll look at you like *you're* the one who's misinformed.

Again, I've been there. Parents who know that they're going to get bullied by their doctor ask if I'll help them so they can push a little further. Then, when they do… suddenly these doctors want to know *who I am* and *why I'm even in the room.*

I've had pediatricians (who at first smiled, shook my hand and welcomed me) turn and then suggest to parents that I should never have been allowed into the exam room to begin with. Not because I was disruptive. But because I knew too much. Because I wasn't playing by the script.

That's the problem. The script is sacred. Step outside it, and the white coat turns defensive.

But if you're a parent who's taken the time to read this book—to understand what true informed consent looks like—you're already ahead. And the next time you walk into a doctor's office, you'll know what kind of doctor you're dealing with. The kind who respects your choices… or the kind who resents them.

Choose wisely.

That's what true informed consent requires. That *before* every injection, the doctor informs the parent of potential side effects—including anaphylaxis, seizures, autoimmune reactions, and yes, death. That they disclose whether long-term safety studies were done. That they explain if a true placebo was used in the trial. That they honestly say: "We don't know how this vaccine will interact with your child's unique physiology. And no, we can't guarantee it's safe."

Unfortunately, that's not how it usually goes down.

Instead, most parents get a 60-second conversation, if that. The doctor walks in, glances at the chart, and says, "Okay, looks like we're due for some shots today." No discussion. No risk disclosure. No time for questions. And if the parent hesitates? Cue the guilt trip.

"Do you want your child to get sick?"

"Are you sure you want to skip this one? These are important."

"This is what the CDC recommends."

They'll repeat slogans like "safe and effective" and "the benefits outweigh the risks," not because they've done a deep dive into the data, but because that's what they were told to say.

Let me put this plainly: when a doctor says "I follow the CDC schedule" or "I recommend the American Academy of Pediatrics protocol," what they're really saying is: "I haven't independently researched this. I'm just passing the buck onto the authorities which I follow."

That's not informed consent. That's blind compliance.

And yet, that's what most parents get. They walk into the exam room expecting the doctor to be an expert on vaccines, only to find out (too late) that the doctor is just a middleman for public health policy.

Want proof? Next time you're in a pediatrician's office, ask this: "Can you guarantee that this vaccine is safe for my child?" "Will you guarantee that my child will not be hurt or even killed by this vaccine?"

They won't say yes. They can't. They'll give you the standard disclaimer: "No drug is 100% safe. But the benefits outweigh the risks."

Ask what those risks are, and they'll cite mild fever, soreness, or rash. Ask about seizures, encephalitis, or autoimmune disorders, and they'll likely brush you off or tell you it's "extremely rare."

But you, dear reader, now know better.

You've read the facts from the studies. You've seen the ingredients. You've followed the logic. You know that adverse events are underreported. You know that $5 billion has been paid out in vaccine injury settlements—and that's just the tip of the iceberg.

You now know more about vaccine science, history, and safety than the average pediatrician. That's not a criticism of your doctor, and it's not an exaggeration. That's a sobering indictment of our medical education system.

Because what's being taught isn't medicine. It's marketing.

When it comes to vaccination, medical schools aren't producing informed practitioners, they're producing obedient implementers. And those implementers are expected to push vaccines as a default, not as an option.

So what does this mean for you as a parent?

It means *you* are now the expert in the room. It means *you* are responsible for asking the hard questions. For demanding the data. For insisting on real informed consent before allowing anything to be injected into your child.

And it means that your right to say "no" is sacred. Legally. Ethically. Morally.[1,2,3]

Because informed consent isn't consent if it's coerced.

It isn't informed if the doctor doesn't know the information.

And it isn't a choice if the only option is compliance.

So the next time you're told, "Your child is due for their shots," stop. Ask. Question. Research. You cannot make an educated decision if you do not have the information to base it on. Isn't your child worth at least that?!

You now have the tools. Use them.

Because no one—not a doctor, not a politician, not a pharmaceutical rep—will ever care more about your child's health than you do.

Chapter Sources

1. U.S. Department of Health and Human Services. (2018). *Informed consent FAQs*. Office for Human Research Protections (OHRP).
2. Beauchamp, T. L., & Childress, J. F. (2019). *Principles of biomedical ethics* (8th ed.). Oxford University Press.
3. American Medical Association. (2016). AMA Code of Medical Ethics: Opinion 2.1.1 – Informed consent. AMA Journal of Ethics.
4. American Medical Association. (2016). *AMA Code of Medical Ethics: Opinion 8.3 – Physicians' responsibilities in disaster response and preparedness*. AMA Journal of Ethics.
5. American Medical Association. (2016). AMA Code of Medical Ethics: Opinion 1.1.2 – Prospective patients. AMA Journal of Ethics.

Chapter 11: Truth #8 - Public School Does *Not* Require Vaccination— Just Exemption Forms

(They're hoping you won't look into it. You should.)

Let's begin with one of the most persistent lies in the entire vaccine debate. You've probably heard it. Maybe you've even repeated it:

"You have to be vaccinated to go to school."

Sounds official, right? Sounds like law. Like some ironclad federal mandate that governs every playground, every classroom, every school bus in America.

Except... it's not true. Not even close.

I don't just say that as someone who's done the research. I say it as someone who's lived it.

Like I mentioned in the introduction to this book—I've never had a single vaccine in my life. Not one. Zero. Nada. And yet, here I am… a doctor.

Now before you think I'm bragging, slow down. This isn't about me. I mention it for one reason: to bust the myth wide open.

You see, I went to K–12 public school. I played dodgeball in gym class, dissected frogs in biology, and got my high school diploma just like everyone else. Then I went to college. A publicly funded college. Earned my undergraduate degree. Then completed postgraduate education and became a licensed doctor.

So, if you really had to "get your shots" to go to school, how exactly did I do it?

Here's the truth: *you don't have to be vaccinated to go to school.* You never have. Not in the way most people think. The requirement is not vaccination. The requirement is *either* vaccination *or* a valid exemption. And every single state offers exemptions.

"But you must be mistaken…"

When I was a kid, and I'd casually mention to people that I wasn't vaccinated, they'd smile politely and say, "Oh, you're just confused. You need shots to go to school."

But I wasn't confused. My parents weren't confused. They knew the laws. They knew that the requirement was not vaccination, but *documentation*—and that documentation could take the form of a vaccine record OR an exemption form.

What the average parent didn't know—because nobody ever told them—was that *you can opt out.*

And I've got the proof.

The Card in My Diploma

At my high school graduation, when I opened the padded diploma case to admire my certificate, something strange caught my eye. Tucked into the corner was a small folded card. At the top, it read: *"Certificate of Immunization."* It had spaces next to each vaccine name, meant for dates, initials, or checkmarks showing compliance with the vaccine schedule.

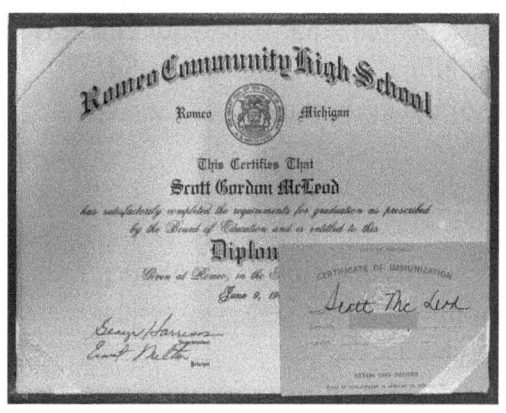

I unfolded it… and every single space was blank.

No dates. No initials. No stamps. Just a handwritten message scrawled across the page in large, unmistakable letters:

"None Given!"

It was like the school nurse wanted to leave me with one final message: "You may have earned your diploma, but you're not getting credit for being vaccinated."

I laughed. Not because it was petty (though it was). I laughed because that little card proved my point better than any argument ever could.

I went to school. I graduated. I never got vaccinated.

So no—vaccines are not required to attend public school.

The Mandate Myth

Here's where the confusion comes in. You hear the word *"mandate,"* and you assume it means *"mandatory."*

But mandates are not unbreakable laws. They're conditional policies.

In fact, neither the federal government nor any state forces a parent to vaccinate their child. What they do is present a choice: "You can comply with the recommended vaccine schedule... OR you can submit an exemption form."

That's not coercion. That's policy cloaked in suggestion—*banking on the hope that you won't question it.*

Most people don't. And that's exactly the way they like it.

The Three Types of Exemptions

Every U.S. state offers *at least one* type of exemption from vaccination. Most offer two. Some offer all three.

Let's break them down.

1. Medical Exemptions
This one's the hardest to get—and the most ironic. A medical exemption is granted when a licensed physician determines that a vaccine would be harmful to the child based on their current health status or history.

In other words: "This vaccine might injure or kill this child, so we're going to exempt them."

Wait… did you catch that?

The very existence of medical exemptions is an admission that *vaccines can harm or kill.*

So if they're dangerous for some, are they really "safe and effective" for all?

Here's the catch: most doctors won't sign off on a medical exemption. Why? Because of the immense pressure put on the medical profession to toe the line. As we discussed in the last chapter, doctors aren't trained to question vaccines. They're trained to promote them.

Even if a doctor understands the risks and respects your right to opt out, they may be unwilling to risk their own license by issuing a medical exemption that goes against the accepted narrative.

So yes, medical exemptions exist. But don't expect them to hand one over with a smile and a clipboard.

2. Religious Exemptions
This is one of the most powerful—and misunderstood—protections in the country.

Millions of Americans object to vaccines based on their deeply held religious, moral, or ethical beliefs.

The First Amendment of the Constitution guarantees freedom of religion. That doesn't just mean the freedom to attend your place of worship. It includes the freedom to make decisions—including medical decisions—based on your religious convictions.

Some religions object to:
- Abortion (many vaccines contain aborted fetal cell lines)
- Cloning and genetic manipulation (used in vaccine production)
- Ingestion or injection of foreign substances (forbidden in some faiths)

And here's the truth: *you don't have to belong to a major religion.* You don't need a letter from your pastor. You don't need to be Catholic, Jewish, Muslim, Mormon, or Amish. You just need to sincerely hold a belief rooted in your moral or religious worldview. That's it.

3. Philosophical Exemptions

Now we're getting into real freedom of thought. Philosophical or *"personal belief"* exemptions are exactly what they sound like. You've reviewed the data. You've thought it through. You don't believe vaccination is right for your child. And so, you opt out. Simple, right?

Except not every state allows this exemption. As of now, about 15 states still honor philosophical exemptions. The rest have chipped away at this freedom in the name of "public health"—even as chronic illness, neurological disorders, and autoimmune diseases continue to rise.

In those 15 states, though, the law still recognizes that you don't need a religion to have a conscience.

You just need to be a thinking, reasoning adult who wants to make an informed decision for your child.

Let's take a closer look at each of the exemption categories in more detail.

First, medical exemptions. These are perhaps the most misunderstood—and most difficult to obtain. They require a licensed physician to provide written documentation stating that a vaccine may be harmful to the child due to a specific medical condition. Sounds reasonable, right? But the catch is that most physicians have been trained to view vaccination as nearly universally safe and effective. The idea that a vaccine could pose a serious risk to an individual is seen as almost blasphemous in many medical circles. That's why, even when a child has a legitimate condition that may warrant exemption, physicians are often reluctant to write it down. They fear professional backlash, possible audits, and in some cases, disciplinary action. So instead of protecting the child, they protect their license. And who suffers? The family.

Next, the religious exemption. This one should be a no-brainer in a country that prides itself on religious freedom. The First Amendment protects not just your right to worship, but your right to live according to your moral and spiritual convictions. For many, that includes the decision not to vaccinate. Whether it's because vaccines contain ingredients derived from aborted fetal tissue, or because they violate beliefs about bodily purity or divine design, or simply because injecting foreign substances into one's body is contrary to their understanding of faith—the religious exemption exists for a reason. And in most states, it doesn't require a letter from your clergy or a theological dissertation. It requires a sincere belief and a simple form.

Then comes the philosophical or personal belief exemption—the one that really gets under the skin of those who want total compliance. Why? Because it acknowledges your right to think, to question, to research, and to decide. It doesn't rely on a medical diagnosis or a religious doctrine. It relies on your informed conscience. The very thing this book is working to empower. Not every state offers this exemption, but for those that do, it's a powerful tool of medical freedom. And it may be the only one left standing if political tides shift further toward coercion.

Of course, many exemption forms include language that allows health departments or schools to exclude your child during an outbreak. That's their loophole. And it's an important one to challenge logically. If vaccines work, *and vaccinated children are protected*, then how does an unvaccinated child pose a threat? If the concern is that the unvaccinated child might catch the illness, isn't that a parental decision? Isn't that the whole point of informed consent?

Once again, we find ourselves back at the heart of the issue: control. Not science. Not logic. Control.

Because if we're being honest, this entire "danger to others" argument falls apart with even a modest amount of critical thinking. Let's walk through it. If your child is fully vaccinated, and you believe that vaccines protect them from disease, then how exactly is my unvaccinated child a risk to yours? Does your vaccine only work when everyone else is vaccinated? Does it magically stop working if there's one unvaccinated kid in the class?

If that's the case, then maybe we need to ask an uncomfortable question: is the problem really the unvaccinated child—or is it that the vaccines themselves aren't as effective as advertised?

That's the dirty little secret no one wants to say out loud. Because once you admit that vaccinated children are still susceptible to the very diseases they were supposedly protected from, you also have to admit that the justification for vaccine mandates completely collapses. It's not about immunity. It's about conformity.

The "dangerous unvaccinated" narrative is a scare tactic. A social weapon. It's used to shame, pressure, and isolate families who don't go along with the program. It's not based on data. It's based on fear.

And let's be honest: if a school is filled with children who are vaccinated, and those vaccines do what they claim to do, then they shouldn't be afraid of the one child who isn't. Unless the real fear is that others might start asking questions too. And that is what the system really fears—not outbreaks, but dissent.

We'll now turn to the current exemption laws in each U.S. state to give you a clearer understanding of where your state stands, and what options you have. Remember: it is your legal right to file an exemption when it is offered—and your moral right to fight for one when it's not.

Let's break this down by state. Because while federal mandates don't exist for school vaccinations, every state has its own system—and its own form of gatekeeping.

All 50 states allow medical exemptions. That's the baseline. But after that, it's a patchwork of rules, politics, and pressure. As of this writing:
- 44 states and Washington D.C. allow religious exemptions.
- 15 states currently allow philosophical or personal belief exemptions.
- Six states—California, New York, Connecticut, Maine, West Virginia and Mississippi—only allow medical exemptions.

Let that sink in. In six U.S. states, your freedom to opt out for personal or religious reasons has been stripped away. And how did that happen? Not because of science. But because of politics, lobbying, and fear-based propaganda.

For the majority of Americans, vaccine exemptions remain your right. But just because it's legal doesn't mean they make it easy. Forms can be hard to find. Language can be intimidating. Some schools may even tell you it's 'not allowed'—until you push back and prove otherwise. But here's the point: you still have the right to opt out. They're hoping you won't look into it. You should.

State Vaccine Exemption Laws

State	Medical	Religious	Philosophical
Alabama	X	X	
Alaska	X	X	X
Arizona	X	X	X
Arkansas	X	X	X
California	X		
Colorado	X	X	X
Connecticut	X		
Delaware	X	X	
Florida	X	X	
Georgia	X	X	
Hawaii	X	X	
Idaho	X	X	X
Illinois	X	X	

Indiana	X	X	
Iowa	X	X	X
Kansas	X	X	X
Kentucky	X	X	
Louisiana	X	X	
Maine	X		
Maryland	X	X	
Massachusetts	X	X	
Michigan	X	X	X
Minnesota	X	X	X
Mississippi	X		
Missouri	X	X	X
Montana	X	X	X
Nebraska	X	X	X
Nevada	X	X	
New Hampshire	X	X	X
New Jersey	X	X	
New Mexico	X	X	
New York	X		
North Carolina	X	X	
North Dakota	X	X	X
Ohio	X	X	

Oklahoma	X	X	X
Oregon	X	X	X
Pennsylvania	X	X	
Rhode Island	X	X	
South Carolina	X	X	
South Dakota	X	X	X
Tennessee	X	X	
Texas	X	X	X
Utah	X	X	X
Vermont	X	X	
Virginia	X	X	
Washington	X	X	X
West Virginia	X		
Wisconsin	X	X	X
Wyoming	X	X	X

What About the Rest of the World?

For the readers who reside outside the US, you may be wondering—what about the rest of the world? Is the "you must be vaccinated to go to school" myth just an American problem? Or is this kind of pressure being felt across the globe?

The short answer? It varies. A lot.

Let's start with Europe. While many European countries *recommend* vaccines, most stop short of making them mandatory. In fact, many EU nations recognize a parent's right to choose whether or not to vaccinate. Countries like the United Kingdom, Sweden, the Netherlands, and Germany (yes, Germany!) do not mandate childhood vaccines for school attendance. They strongly recommend them, sure—but there are no criminal penalties, no school bans, and no government agents knocking on doors with needles. In the Netherlands, they even have one of the highest rates of vaccine skepticism in Europe—and guess what? They're still functioning just fine.

Then there are countries like Italy, France, and Poland, where mandates do exist, but enforcement varies wildly. Italy, for instance, went through a period of tightening mandates under political pressure... only to loosen them again due to backlash. France currently mandates a list of 11 vaccines for children—on paper. But in practice, there are still routes of resistance, and a robust community of medical freedom advocates continues to push back.

Now let's look east.

In Asia, things can get a little more heavy-handed. China has strict vaccine compliance policies, and questioning government vaccination programs is not exactly encouraged. In countries like Japan, however, while vaccines are recommended, they've had a rocky history—especially after lawsuits involving vaccine injuries in the 1980's and '90s. As a result, Japan has adopted a more cautious approach, and parental consent remains central to their vaccine programs.

Even in Australia and New Zealand, countries often cited for their "public health discipline," vaccine mandates aren't as cut and dry as they seem. Australia has implemented what they call the "No Jab, No Pay" and "No Jab, No Play" policies—essentially coercion-by-wallet. You can technically say no, but the government might withhold childcare benefits or daycare access. That's not medical freedom. That's financial blackmail dressed up as public health policy.

So what's the pattern?

Around the world, governments vary in how they push vaccines, but the pattern is always the same: Pressure. Whether it's school enrollment, financial penalties, or social shaming, they try to make opting out as uncomfortable as possible.

But here's the universal truth: In nearly every country, *there are paths to exemption.* You just have to dig for them. Religious and philosophical exemptions might be more common in the U.S., but medical exemptions are available in most parts of the world. The key is knowing your rights, learning the law in your country or region, and pushing back when that law is twisted or ignored.

The idea that "you have no choice" is not just a myth, it's a lie. Whether you're in the States or halfway across the world, medical freedom is still your right. You just have to be willing to stand up and claim it.

At the end of the day, this chapter isn't just about school policies. It's about freedom. It's about informed decisions. It's about being the parent, the guardian, the person who gets to say what goes into your child's body.

They want you to believe the law is black and white. It's not. They want you to think you have no say. You do. And once you realize that, once you stand up and use that knowledge, you can never go back to blindly complying again.

Because once you see the fine print, the exemption forms, the loopholes, the truth—you can't unsee it.

And if you don't believe this is a fight for control, just consider this: in the summer of 2025, the American Academy of Pediatrics publicly announced that they are strongly recommending the elimination of both philosophical and religious vaccination exemptions for school attendance for ALL states. Translation? They don't trust you to make medical decisions for your own child. They don't have your family's best interests at heart—they have their agenda. They, along with the doctors who follow their marching orders, want full control over what goes into your child's body. Your beliefs? Irrelevant. Your values? Disposable. Your rights? Negotiable—unless you stand up and defend them.

And here's the truth they hope you'll never realize: once philosophical and religious exemptions are gone, there's no going back. Medical exemptions are already being strangled to the point of uselessness—approved only in the most extreme, government-approved cases. If you let them take away these last protections, your child's medical decisions will no longer belong to you. They will belong to the state, the pharmaceutical companies, and the institutions that profit from compliance. This is why you must pay attention—not just in the doctor's office, but in your state legislature, your school boards, and your voting booth. Your right to say "no" is not self-sustaining—it's only alive as long as you fight for it.

    We're not done yet. There's more to uncover. More truth to expose. So let's keep going.

Chapter 12: Truth #9 - Unvaccinated Children Are Often Healthier Than Their Peers

(The data is inconvenient—but it's there.)

I've never had a vaccine in my life.

I say that not to gloat, not to start a fight, and certainly not to court controversy. I say it because it's true—and because it flies directly in the face of one of the most stubbornly held beliefs in modern society: that vaccines are what keep children healthy. That without them, kids will drop like flies from every sniffle, sneeze, and sore throat. That vaccination is the wall between order and chaos, between a healthy life and a crippled one. I'm living proof that isn't true.

So are my children. So are my siblings. So are their children, and their children's children.

We were all raised without vaccines. Not "under-vaccinated." Not "delayed schedule." Not "just a few." None. Zero. Zilch. And guess what? We survived. Not only that, we thrived.

Growing up in the 1970s, being unvaccinated was almost unheard of. My parents were the unicorns of the PTA, the ones who filled out the exemption form instead of the vaccine card. When I'd mention to friends or teachers that I'd never been vaccinated, I'd get the same look people give when you say you've never seen Star Wars. A strange mix of awe and suspicion. Most people didn't believe me. They'd insist I must be mistaken. That I *had* to have had *some* shots, because "you can't go to school if you're not vaccinated."

And yet, there I was—on the playground, in the classroom, walking across the graduation stage with a diploma in hand—completely unvaccinated.

But more importantly, I wasn't sick. In fact, I was *healthier* than most of my classmates. I missed fewer days of school. I bounced back quicker when I *did* get sick. I didn't have asthma, food allergies, chronic ear infections, or neurological problems. As I grew older, that trend continued. My health was not some stroke of luck—it was a pattern. And that pattern held across my family. My siblings were the same way. Our children—unvaccinated like us—showed the same robust, bounce-back, energy-charged health that people now wistfully describe as "how kids used to be."

The Missing Study

For decades, we've been asking one very simple question: Why hasn't there ever been a large-scale, gold-standard, controlled study comparing vaccinated vs. unvaccinated children's health outcomes? The standard answer? "Because it would be unethical to leave children unprotected." Let that sink in. They refuse to do the study—not because it's impossible, not because it's impractical, but because it's already assumed that the unvaccinated kids would fare worse. That's not science. That's circular logic wrapped in a lab coat.

But even that excuse is falling apart. Today, there are millions of unvaccinated children in the United States alone. The population is large enough, diverse enough, and trackable enough to run countless studies. And yet—crickets. Why? Because the results wouldn't just challenge the narrative. They would obliterate it.

Let's go beyond my family's experience and take a serious look at one of the most fascinating case studies available in America today: the *Amish*. If you've ever spent any time in or around Amish communities, you'll notice something that doesn't quite fit with the narrative we're so often sold. These are people who choose to live without the conveniences of modern medicine, who raise their children without vaccinations—and yet, somehow, they aren't dropping like flies.

Let's be honest. If vaccines were as essential to survival as we've been told, the Amish should be an extinct people by now. But they're not. In fact, they're thriving in their own quiet, deliberate way. They don't just reject vaccines—they reject most forms of modern medicine entirely. So where's the epidemic? Where are the body piles? Where are the overflowing hospitals and quarantine zones?

They don't exist. What does exist, however, is an astounding lack of chronic illness. Rates of autism in the Amish community, for example, are staggeringly low. And I don't mean "a little bit lower." I mean *near non-existent*. In fact, in 2005, a mainstream journalist named

Dan Olmsted from UPI went looking for cases of autism among the Amish in Lancaster County, Pennsylvania. He couldn't find any. Not one. The CDC's own data says that nationally, autism affects 1 in every 36 children today.[2] Among the Amish? Olmsted identified only three cases in a population of thousands—and at least two of those children had been vaccinated.[1]

Coincidence? Critics will immediately shout, "Correlation isn't causation!" And yes, they're technically right. That's an inductive argument, and it doesn't prove causation. But here's the catch: when the research—that would move it through a deductive process and certainty—is deliberately avoided, denied, or suppressed, we have to start asking *why*. If science were truly objective and transparent, wouldn't this be worth exploring? Wouldn't the health of the Amish raise serious questions? Wouldn't this be the perfect unvaccinated control group?

Instead of digging deeper, mainstream science shrugs its shoulders and walks away. No studies. No follow-ups. Just silence. And that silence speaks volumes.

Now, let's look at the broader health picture. The Amish have extremely low rates of asthma, allergies, diabetes, autoimmune diseases, and cancer compared to the general population.[3,4,5,6] They eat whole foods, work physically demanding jobs, live in clean rural environments, and yes, they reject most pharmaceuticals. But it's hard to untangle these variables precisely because no one wants to actually study them. That's not an accident—it's a strategy. Because if a large-scale, peer-reviewed, vaccinated-vs-unvaccinated health study were ever conducted using the Amish as a control group, the results would be catastrophic for the vaccine narrative.

So why don't we hear about this? Simple. Because it's inconvenient.

Because the vaccine program isn't a neutral science project. It's a multibillion-dollar juggernaut backed by government mandates, media partnerships, and corporate lobbying. If it were ever shown—really shown—that unvaccinated children tend to be healthier, that the diseases they're supposedly protected from are less deadly than the treatments themselves, the entire system would collapse.

We can't have that now, can we?

So instead, the narrative soldiers on. And those of us who grew up unvaccinated—those of us raising our children the same way—we're treated like outliers, like we somehow lucked out and dodged the bullet.

But it wasn't luck.

It was informed choice. It was medical freedom. It was trusting in the body, not the needle.

But let's not stop there. Let's travel even farther back and farther away to one of the most astonishing populations the world has ever seen: the Hunzakuts of Northern Pakistan.

Tucked away in the mountainous borderlands near China and Afghanistan, the Hunza people have lived in peaceful seclusion for centuries. If there was ever a real-world example of the phrase "untouched by modern civilization," the Hunza fit the bill.

No cars. No processed food. No pharmaceutical products. No vaccines. And yet, somehow, their life expectancy extended well into their 100s—some to 110, 120, even older. That's not internet lore—that's been documented and reported by doctors and explorers since the early 20th century.[7,8,9,10]

Their secret? It wasn't a secret at all. Their lifestyle was built on fresh, local, organic produce, glacial water, fermented foods, mountain air, and constant physical activity. They ate apricot kernels, sprouted grains, and drank from streams rich in minerals. Their children played outside barefoot, building natural immunity from birth. Their medicine was food, and their doctors were their elders.

Western doctors who visited the Hunza in the early 1900s—such as Dr. Robert McCarrison—reported astonishingly low rates of disease. No cancer. No diabetes. No obesity. No heart disease. And again, no vaccines. When these people did get sick, it was mild and short-lived. Their bodies were resilient, their immune systems robust.[7]

But here's the plot twist. Since the introduction of modern western medicine, including vaccines, into the Hunza Valley in the mid-to-late 20th century, their health statistics have changed. Processed food made its way in. Medical clinics appeared. And yes—vaccines were introduced. Today, the average Hunza lifespan is estimated to be closer to 70 or 80… just like ours. Not the mythic longevity they once had. Their story serves as a living, breathing contrast between a naturally healthy society and one shaped by pharmaceutical "progress."

Again, critics will scoff, "Correlation isn't causation!" And again, we say: then do the research! But they won't. Because the results would be inconvenient. They would challenge the status quo. And worst of all, they might make people think for themselves.

Modern Science's Favorite Escape Hatch: "Too Many Variables"

Whenever a conversation starts to lean toward uncomfortable truths—especially those that challenge pharmaceutical dogma—you'll hear the same tired phrase: "There are too many variables."

That's the fallback. The smoke bomb. The intellectual escape hatch.

Ask why we don't have large-scale, peer-reviewed studies comparing vaccinated and unvaccinated populations, and you'll get this hand-wringing answer: "Well, there are so many lifestyle differences between groups like the Amish and the general population—it would be impossible to draw valid conclusions."

Translation? "We don't want to look."

Let's imagine for a moment that the tables were turned. That there was a remote, isolated population somewhere with sky-high vaccine uptake and nearly nonexistent rates of chronic disease, neurological disorders, and developmental delay. Would the public health machine dismiss them with a shrug and say, "Too many variables"? Of course not. They'd fund entire research institutes to figure out how to replicate those results. They'd be on every news broadcast, every morning show, every TED Talk.

But when the health outcomes contradict the narrative—when unvaccinated people seem to be thriving, not dying—suddenly we're not interested in science anymore. Suddenly, the same people who chant "follow the science" would rather follow the silence.

This is not about intellectual integrity. It's about preserving a paradigm. It's about control.

While the mainstream likes to pretend no comparative data exists, a handful of independent researchers and organizations have dared to ask the forbidden question: Are unvaccinated children actually healthier?

And wouldn't you know—it turns out they often are.

In 2020, Dr. James Lyons-Weiler and Dr. Paul Thomas (a board-certified pediatrician) published a peer-reviewed study comparing vaccinated and unvaccinated children in Dr. Thomas's Oregon practice over a ten-year span. The study was meticulous. It used patient medical records, controlled for confounders, and asked a basic question: how did health outcomes differ?

The results? The unvaccinated children had significantly lower rates of allergies, asthma, ear infections, behavioral issues, and developmental delays. In fact, the longer a child remained unvaccinated, the healthier they tended to be.[11]

The response? Not applause. Not engagement. Not open debate. No—Dr. Thomas had his medical license suspended within days of the study's publication. It was Dr. Wakefield all over again, and it was a message to every other physician who might dare to follow in his footsteps: don't even think about it!

The message wasn't subtle. It was a warning shot.

You can't say vaccines make children healthier without data.

But apparently, you also can't say vaccines make children sicker even if you have the data.

Ask parents of children with autism, and you'll hear a hauntingly familiar story: "He was developing normally… and then something changed." Often, the change came after a routine pediatric visit. The kind with multiple injections. The kind where doctors told them, "Don't worry, it's safe. Just a little fever."

That's not a conspiracy theory. That's a pattern. And it's a pattern that's shown up thousands upon thousands of times—in kitchens, in therapy rooms, in Facebook groups filled with shell-shocked moms and dads trying to make sense of what happened to their once-healthy child.

For decades, the medical establishment has insisted there's "no link" between vaccines and autism. That phrase has been repeated so many times it might as well be a hypnotic chant. But what happens when actual data gets in the way of that narrative?

Let's talk about the **Mawson and Jacob (2025)** study—a peer-reviewed paper that dropped like a bomb in the world of public health research.[14]

This study examined a nationally representative sample of *over 11,000* nine-year-old children enrolled in Medicaid, focusing on the connection between vaccination and neurodevelopmental disorders. Not a small sample. Not anecdotal. This was a real-world look at real children—exactly the kind of research the CDC always says we don't have.

And the findings? Let's just say they were *inconvenient*.

The researchers found that *vaccinated children were significantly more likely to be diagnosed with autism, ADHD, and developmental delays* compared to their unvaccinated peers. In fact, they found that the odds of having one or more neurodevelopmental disorders were *more than three to four times higher in vaccinated children.* Three to four times.

The paper stated:

> "Based on the records of 47,155 children enrolled in the Florida Medicaid program from 1999 to 2011, the results of this study provide evidence of significant associations between visits for vaccinations and diagnoses of neurodevelopmental disorders (NDDs). Vaccinated children were significantly more likely than the unvaccinated to have been diagnosed with ASD, hyperkinetic syndrome, learning disorders, epilepsy or seizures, encephalopathy, and tic disorders, with odds ratios ranging from 2.7 for ASD, 5.2 for encephalopathy, and 6.3 for tic disorders.".[14]

It went on to point out the increased risk of Autism Spectrum Disorder (ASD) increased with the number of vaccination visits:

> *"Increasing numbers of vaccinations were associated with significantly increased risks of ASD. Children with just one vaccination visit were 1.7 times more likely to have been diagnosed with ASD than the unvaccinated, whereas those with 11 or more visits were 4.4 times more likely to have been diagnosed with ASD than those with no visit. The increasing risk of ASD associated with numbers of visits for vaccinations suggests that some component or components of vaccines have progressively adverse effects."*[14]

If vaccines have nothing to do with autism—or any other neurodevelopmental disorder for that matter—then why did this study uncover such a stark difference? Why did the unvaccinated group come out on top across every category of neurological health?

The authors of the study didn't claim vaccines cause autism outright. They weren't pushing an agenda. They simply did what good scientists are supposed to do: they looked at the data. And the data said loud and clear that *there's a serious correlation here*—one that deserves much deeper investigation.

But don't hold your breath. The mainstream media didn't touch it. The CDC didn't issue a press release. Your pediatrician didn't bring it up at your child's next check-up.

Because acknowledging these findings would mean pulling back the curtain on one of the most sacred cows in modern medicine. And that, apparently, is a bigger threat than autism itself.

Let's put it plainly: the Mawson study adds another loud, glaring warning siren to the conversation that too many health officials are desperate to silence. It confirms what countless parents have been shouting from the rooftops: *something's not right here*. And if the vaccine schedule really is safe and effective, it shouldn't require silencing scientists and ignoring inconvenient data to keep that illusion intact.

And Let's Not Forget the Elephant in the Exam Room: Chronic Illness in Kids

Look around at the average American child today. Go to a public playground. Sit in on a kindergarten class. Talk to an elementary school teacher. Ask a pediatric nurse what's changed in the last 30 years.

They'll all tell you the same thing: we are raising the sickest generation of children in modern history.

More than half of U.S. children now suffer from at least one chronic condition. One in five has a diagnosed developmental delay.[12,13]

Food allergies are everywhere. ADHD is exploding. Asthma inhalers and EpiPens are part of the school supplies list. And nobody seems to be asking why.

We're told it's "just better diagnostics." That we're "more aware" now.

No. That's a cop-out. Kids used to bring PB&J to school without killing anyone. A hyper kid in the 80s got a note sent home, not a prescription. A peanut allergy was rare enough to be a trivia question.

Now it's a crisis. And the common factor that's scaled with that crisis? The childhood vaccine schedule.

Since 1986—when pharmaceutical companies were given legal immunity for vaccine injuries—the number of recommended vaccines for children has skyrocketed. So has chronic illness. That's not a coincidence. That's a correlation begging to be investigated. But it won't be. Because the implications are too damning.

Instead, they blame genetics. As if human DNA mutated sometime around the Reagan administration.

"Correlation Isn't Causation"—Unless It's Convenient

Let's take a moment to talk about one of the laziest, most abused phrases in the entire scientific playbook. One that I've already referred to several times in this book: "correlation isn't causation."

Yes, that's true. Correlation alone doesn't prove cause and effect. It's a foundational principle of science.

But here's the dirty little secret: when it fits the narrative, correlation is treated like gospel. When vaccine uptake goes up and a disease incidence goes down, it's immediately hailed as proof of vaccine effectiveness—even if no double-blind controlled study was ever done. But when you flip the lens—when you point out that chronic illness rises in lockstep with vaccine uptake—suddenly, correlation is meaningless.

That's not how real science works.

In science, correlations are clues. They guide us toward questions that need answering. They provide patterns that call for hypothesis, experimentation, and analysis. They are tools that can lead us from inductive theories to deductive facts.

But if the research that would allow us to move from correlation to causation is never conducted—if it's actively discouraged, defunded, or censored—then the claim "correlation isn't causation" becomes a form of intellectual gaslighting.

You're not allowed to ask. And when you do, you're told you haven't proven anything. That's not science. That's manipulation.

The Inconvenient Truth They Don't Want You to See

So here we are. After an entire chapter (and a lifetime of living outside the pharmaceutical bubble) we're left with a question that's as pressing as ever: *Where are the studies?*

We've heard the excuse ad nauseam: "Correlation isn't causation." It's the intellectual equivalent of plugging your ears and yelling *la la la* when confronted with evidence that doesn't fit the narrative. And yes, technically, that's true. Correlation alone doesn't prove causation. But it does tell you where to look. It's a red flag. A signal flare. A blinking neon sign that says, *"Hey, something interesting is happening here—dig deeper!"*

But the digging never happens.

Why? Because the powers that be don't want the truth unearthed. They don't want a scientific reckoning with the real-life outcomes of the unvaccinated. They don't want side-by-side comparisons of children raised with every CDC-recommended injection against those raised with none. Because when you start comparing—when you actually open your eyes and look—you begin to see what many of us have known all along: unvaccinated children are, in many cases, healthier than their vaccinated peers.

They have fewer chronic illnesses. Fewer developmental delays. Fewer allergies. Fewer neurological issues. They miss fewer days of school. They bounce back faster from routine illness. And they carry none of the toxic burden of aluminum, formaldehyde, polysorbate 80, or aborted fetal cell fragments that come with today's vaccines.

And no, that's not just anecdotal. It's observable. It's replicable. It's verifiable in communities like the Amish and the Hunzakuts. It's showing up in families across the country and around the world who are saying, *"No, thank you"* to pharmaceutical dependency and choosing instead to trust in the body's design. They're not conspiracy theorists. They're not reckless. They're not dangerous.

They're healthy.

They're thriving.

And they're growing in number.

Millions of parents today are choosing not to vaccinate. And far from being the fringe minority that the media tries to portray, they are teachers, lawyers, nurses, small business owners, engineers, athletes, and yes—doctors. They've done the research. They've read the science. They've seen the data. And they've watched what happens when kids are raised without a shot in sight.

These families aren't living in fear. They're not wringing their hands about measles or RSV. They're living boldly, raising strong, resilient children with immune systems that were designed to adapt, respond, and recover. They're proof that the *"unvaccinated = unsafe"* narrative isn't just wrong—it's lazy. And the more we silence the lived experiences of these families, the more we bury the very evidence that could transform public health for the better.

But maybe that's the point.

Because once you see it, once you see the cracks in the story, you can't unsee them. Once you meet a healthy, vibrant, never-been-vaccinated child, you realize how much of what we've been sold is just that: *a sales pitch.*

The vaccine program, for all its glossy brochures and smiling cartoon syringes, can't answer this one nagging question: If vaccines are so essential to health, then why are so many of the unvaccinated doing just fine—better, even—without them?

That's not a question they want you to ask.

But we're asking it anyway.

And we're not alone.

In the next chapter of this book, we'll tackle one last lingering misconception: that those of us who question vaccines must be crazy. That we're fringe. Anti-science. Irresponsible. Dangerous. That we've fallen down some rabbit hole of misinformation and can't find our way back out.

No. Not even close.

The truth is, people who say no to vaccines aren't crazy—they're paying attention.

They've read the fine print. They've connected the dots. And they've chosen the path of critical thinking, caution, and courage. In Chapter 13, we'll dive into what it really means to be vaccine-hesitant in a world that punishes independent thought—and why that hesitation just might be the most rational choice of all.

Because if you've made it this far in the book, odds are, you're not crazy either.

You're just waking up.

And once you do, there's no going back.

Chapter Sources

1. Olmsted, D. (2005, January 9). *The Amish anomaly*. United Press International.
2. Centers for Disease Control and Prevention. (2023). *Data and statistics on autism spectrum disorder*. U.S. Department of Health & Human Services.
3. Von Mutius, E., Vercelli, D., Farm Studies Consortium. (2010). Farm living: effects on childhood asthma and allergy. *Nature Reviews Immunology, 10*(12), 861–868.
4. Stein, M. M., Hrusch, C. L., Gozdz, J., Igartua, C., Pivniouk, V., Murray, S. E., ... & Ober, C. (2016). Innate immunity and asthma risk in Amish and Hutterite farm children. *New England Journal of Medicine, 375*(5), 411–421.
5. Miller, F. D., & Brann, A. W. (2006). The health status of the Amish: A review of the literature. *Journal of Multicultural Nursing & Health, 12*(3), 44–48.
6. Huff, K. (2015). Amish and cancer: A case of low incidence. *Journal of Community Health Nursing, 32*(4), 211–217.
7. McCarrison, R. (1921). *Studies in deficiency disease*. London: Henry Frowde and Hodder & Stoughton.
8. Bottomley, M. (1960). *Hunza: The Himalayan Shangri-La*. London: Cassell & Company Ltd.
9. Robinson, J. I. (1963). The Hunza: Lost kingdom of the Himalayas. New York: Funk & Wagnalls.
10. Szekely, E. (1972). The Essene health and longevity program. Marina del Rey, CA: Academy Books.
11. Lyons-Weiler, J., & Thomas, P. (2020). Relative incidence of office visits and cumulative rates of billed diagnoses along the axis of

vaccination. *International Journal of Environmental Research and Public Health, 17*(22), 8674.
12. Zablotsky, B., Black, L. I., Maenner, M. J., Schieve, L. A., Danielson, M. L., Bitsko, R. H., & Blumberg, S. J. (2019). Prevalence and trends of developmental disabilities among children in the United States: 2009–2017. *Pediatrics, 144*(4), e20190811.
13. Bethell, C. D., Kogan, M. D., Strickland, B. B., Schor, E. L., Robertson, J., & Newacheck, P. W. (2011). A national and state profile of leading health problems and health care quality for US children: Key insurance disparities and across-state variations. *Academic Pediatrics, 11*(3), S22–S33.
14. Mawson A R., Jacob B. Vaccination and Neurodevelopmental Disorders: A Study of Nine-Year-Old Children Enrolled in Medicaid. Science, Public Health Policy and the Law. 2025 Jan 23; v6.2019-2025

Chapter 13: Truth #10 - People Who Say No to Vaccines Aren't Crazy— They're Paying Attention

(They've read the fine print. You should too.)

Let's get something straight right from the start.

People who say no to vaccines are not crazy.

They're not reckless. They're not stupid. They're not selfish. And they're definitely not "anti-science."

In fact, more often than not, they're some of the most well-informed, well-researched, and medically literate people you'll ever meet. These aren't conspiracy theorists living in the woods with tinfoil hats and bunker rations. These are educated, thoughtful individuals who have dared to ask questions that most people are too afraid—or too conditioned—to ask.

You're reading this book, so chances are, you're one of them. Or you're on your way to becoming one. Either way, welcome to the club. It's not a cult. It's not a fringe movement. It's simply a group of people who've read the fine print.

And realized something doesn't add up.

Because here's what I know from decades of personal experience: the overwhelming majority of people who choose not to vaccinate didn't start out that way. They started where most people do —trusting the system. Believing that doctors always know best. Believing that public health agencies have no agenda. Believing that pharmaceutical companies are in it for the greater good.

Then something happened. A conversation. A reaction. A story that didn't fit the script. A moment that cracked open the door just wide enough to let in a question. And from there? A cascade of investigation. Reading. Listening. Digging. Connecting dots. Realizing just how much of what we've been told is marketing dressed up as medicine.

That's the part no one wants to talk about. The "anti-vaxxers" aren't the ones blindly following anyone. They're the ones who stopped. They're the ones who hit pause and said, "Wait a minute… something's off here."

Meanwhile, the ones throwing stones—calling names, mocking, dismissing—are often the least informed in the room. They parrot headlines. They regurgitate slogans. They don't know the ingredients in a single vaccine, but they're positive you're wrong for questioning them.

It's ironic, isn't it? The people calling you uneducated are the ones who've never spent a single hour studying the topic. But you? You've spent dozens. Hundreds. Maybe even thousands.

Like I have.

As I stated before, I've spent the last 35+ years researching vaccines. Not casually. Not just scrolling through headlines. I mean reading government documents, court transcripts, clinical trial data, peer-reviewed studies, vaccine package inserts, and medical textbooks. I've sat through lectures, listened to whistleblowers, interviewed parents, and watched the evolution of the childhood vaccine schedule go from "a few shots" to "how many syringes can we fit into one visit?"

I didn't get paid to do this. I didn't have a research grant. No pharmaceutical company sent me a thank-you check. I did it because I had to. Because when you start seeing what's behind the curtain, you can't unsee it.

Meanwhile, your average pediatrician has never even read a vaccine insert.

Let me say that again: your doctor—the person giving you advice on vaccines—has never read the actual product insert for the shots they're injecting into children's bodies. They don't know that the insert says *"has not been evaluated for carcinogenic or mutagenic potential."* They don't know that seizure, Guillain-Barré syndrome, or autoimmune disease are listed as "possible adverse events." They don't know that some vaccines are made with fetal cell lines or animal DNA.

They just know what they were told in a lecture or what came down the pipeline from the CDC.

And most of them never question it.

Why? Because their education taught them not to. Because questioning the medical consensus is frowned upon—punished even. Because for all the pomp and circumstance of a medical degree, it often comes with a collar and a leash.

That's the real difference between the average healthcare consumer and those who choose not to vaccinate: *critical thinking.*

People who say no have done their homework. They've read the footnotes. They've followed the money. They've listened to parents—not just experts in white coats. They've wrestled with the hard questions and come out the other side with clarity.

And let's not kid ourselves. It takes courage to go against the grain. To have the entire media, school system, and medical establishment telling you that you're endangering your child and still say, "I've made my decision."

That's not ignorance. That's integrity. That's parenting.

And as more people wake up—more parents, more professionals, even more physicians—this movement isn't slowing down. It's growing. Because truth resonates. Once people hear it, once they see it, it's almost impossible to un-hear or un-see.

So here, we'll take a closer look at just who some of these "crazy" people really are—doctors, scientists, immunologists, medical professionals—who've looked at the same data you have and reached the same conclusion: It's not that we're uninformed. It's that we're paying attention.

Let's talk about the "crazy" people.

You know, the ones who spent their lives in colleges, earned advanced degrees, held prestigious positions, and then—somewhere along the way—*dared* to question the holy grail of modern medicine: the vaccine.

These aren't basement bloggers or "Facebook researchers." These are board-certified, peer-reviewed, published, tenured professionals. And they didn't speak out because it was convenient.

Most of them spoke out knowing full well what it would cost them—reputation, position, funding, even their medical licenses. But they did it anyway. Why? Because truth has a nasty habit of demanding to be spoken.

And let's not forget some of the most intelligent, credentialed people who have stood tall in the face of the medical machine. These aren't basement bloggers or angry internet trolls. These are professionals—experts—who've put their names, reputations, and careers on the line because they saw something that didn't add up, and they refused to stay quiet. People like:

Dr. Robert Mendelsohn, who was a pediatrician, professor at the University of Illinois, and a best-selling author of books like *Confessions of a Medical Heretic*. He didn't mince words. He called the modern medical system "religious medicine" and warned parents about the blind trust they place in pediatricians who follow vaccine schedules like gospel. He wrote extensively about how vaccines were neither as safe nor as effective as advertised—and this was *decades ago*.

Dr. Suzanne Humphries, a board-certified nephrologist (kidney doctor), began questioning vaccines after seeing patients suffer kidney failure following vaccinations—often after no other risk factors. She did what good doctors are supposed to do: she asked questions. She reviewed the data. And the deeper she looked, the worse it got. She now speaks internationally, challenging the narrative with meticulously sourced, data-rich presentations that mainstream medicine refuses to address.

Dr. Larry Palevsky, a New York pediatrician with impeccable credentials, began asking the same basic question we asked in the last chapter: Why aren't we studying the health of vaccinated vs. unvaccinated children? When he started noticing patterns—more ear infections, more allergies, more asthma, more developmental delays in vaccinated kids—he began to speak out. He was blacklisted. Not because he was wrong, but because he refused to shut up.

Dr. Sherri Tenpenny, an osteopathic physician, has dissected every vaccine on the childhood schedule and can quote their ingredients and adverse effects chapter and verse. She's become a target of the media precisely because she knows what she's talking about.

Dr. Michael Yeadon, former Pfizer Vice President and Chief Science Officer for allergy and respiratory research, has become one of the most outspoken critics of the pharmaceutical industry's overreach, especially in the vaccine realm. When someone who helped run Pfizer's science division starts ringing alarm bells—you'd think people might want to listen.

Dr. Tetyana Obukhanych, a PhD immunologist trained at Harvard and Stanford, turned heads when she began publicly speaking out about the gaps and myths in the mainstream understanding of immunity and vaccination. Her open letter to legislators has become a foundational piece of advocacy.

Dr. Yehuda Shoenfeld, often referred to as the "father of autoimmunology," has published over 2,000 scientific papers and edited over 30 books on the immune system. He is perhaps best known in vaccine circles for his work on Autoimmune/Inflammatory Syndrome Induced by Adjuvants (ASIA)—a condition now linked to vaccine components like aluminum.

Del Bigtree, a former Emmy-winning producer for *The Doctors* and *Dr. Phil*, left mainstream television to create *The HighWire*, a media platform dedicated to exposing vaccine science corruption and defending informed consent. He's sharp, relentless, and widely followed for good reason.

Robert F. Kennedy, Jr.—now Secretary of Health and Human Services, but long before that, a presidential candidate, attorney, and founder of Children's Health Defense—has been one of the most consistent and fearless voices in exposing conflicts of interest within the vaccine industry. He's been vilified for daring to ask tough questions, but he's never wavered.

Aaron Siri, Esq. – An attorney who has become one of the foremost legal voices in the battle for vaccine transparency and medical freedom. As managing partner of Siri & Glimstad LLP, he has represented countless individuals, families, and organizations in landmark cases challenging vaccine mandates, defending informed consent, and demanding the release of hidden safety data from pharmaceutical companies and government agencies. Siri has also appeared before Congress and written extensively about the legal and ethical implications of forced vaccination. He is the author of *Vaccines, Amen: The Religion of Vaccines*, a powerful examination of how blind faith and institutional loyalty have replaced evidence and accountability in modern medicine. His tireless advocacy has made him both a champion for truth and a thorn in the side of the pharmaceutical establishment.

Greg Glaser, Esq., a California attorney, has gone to battle for medical freedom in courtrooms across the country. He helped author the landmark Control Group litigation and has fought tirelessly to preserve vaccine choice in a hostile legal climate.

Patricia Finn, Esq., often called "The Good Health Lawyer," has represented families across the country in vaccine injury and exemption cases. She's fearless in defending parents who dare to say no—and she knows the law inside and out.

And then there's **Dr. Andrew Wakefield**. The media made him the poster child for vaccine heresy—turning his name into a punchline. But how many people know that he never said vaccines caused autism?

That his now-infamous study merely suggested a possible *association* between the MMR vaccine and gastrointestinal symptoms in children with autism, and that it called for *more research*? That 12 other physicians co-authored that paper? That most of them never retracted the findings? That Wakefield was targeted not because he was a fraud, but because he was a threat?

These are not fringe loonies. These are highly intelligent people—people with stethoscopes, lab coats, and law degrees who once believed in the vaccine program—until the evidence pulled them in a different direction. And the moment they stepped out of line, the machine turned on them.

And let's be clear—this is a *very* short list of the extremely intelligent, credentialed, thoughtful professionals who have taken a stand. There are hundreds—*thousands*—more out there. Scientists, researchers, nurses, teachers, therapists, and parents with advanced degrees who have read the fine print and refused to blindly comply.

And then—there are the everyday citizens. People just like you. They're not on TV. They don't have titles or platforms. But they've done their homework. They've stayed up late reading vaccine inserts, scrolling through PubMed studies, dissecting VAERS data, and digging through government reports that most people will never touch. They've watched friends or family suffer after "routine" shots. They've sat in pediatrician offices asking questions no one wanted to answer. These people are not ignorant. They're not reckless. They're not conspiracy theorists. They're informed. Deeply informed.

They are the parents, teachers, nurses, engineers, mechanics, farmers, small business owners—regular people who took the time to look into what they were being told. And they saw the red flags. They connected the dots. They saw the fine print that others ignored—and it changed them. Forever. They aren't famous. Many will never be invited to speak on a stage. But they're out there, and they're growing in number. They're reading, questioning, organizing, and educating. Quietly, relentlessly, and with fierce integrity.

But here's the part that should fire you up: They're not backing down. And neither are we.

We're not the ones blindly following orders. We're not the ones parroting talking points. We're not the ones gaslighting parents who just want answers. We're the ones doing the reading. We're the ones asking the inconvenient questions. We're the ones digging through the fine print, reading the actual inserts, following the money, listening to the injured, and demanding accountability.

We're not "anti-science."

We are precisely what science is supposed to look like—curious, critical, and courageous.

This movement—this global awakening—isn't built on conspiracy theories. It's built on evidence, lived experience, medical malpractice, whistleblowers, data, grief, truth, and the undeniable power of asking "why?"

So the next time someone calls you crazy, smile and say: "No, I've just read the fine print. Have you?"

So here we are. Thirteen chapters in, and if you've made it this far, you've proven the very point this chapter set out to make: you're not crazy. You're not irresponsible. You're not some reckless renegade putting your kids in danger. You are what every parent should aspire to be—*informed*.

You didn't get here by accident. You got here because something didn't sit right. Maybe it was a gut feeling. Maybe it was a story you heard. Maybe it was your own experience. Or maybe it was simply that you refused to outsource your critical thinking to the same institutions that told you margarine was healthy, cigarettes were safe, and opioids were good medicine.

Whatever it was, you paused. You questioned. You researched. And you ended up here.

And that *matters*.

Because the world needs more people who don't just "go along to get along." The world needs people who are willing to pull the thread and see what unravels. Who refuse to ignore the inconsistencies. Who recognize that being "pro-health" doesn't mean being pro-injection.

We've been told for decades that people who refuse vaccines are fringe lunatics. Irresponsible. Dangerous. Unscientific. But here's what that really means: you didn't listen to your master. You didn't take your seat at the back of the classroom and keep your mouth shut. You didn't read the script they gave you. You read *everything else* instead. You read the package inserts, the published studies, the VAERS reports, the whistleblower testimony, the court transcripts. You read the fine print.

And when you read the fine print, you realized something chilling: The people who are supposed to protect you aren't doing their jobs. The agencies that say they're independent aren't. The doctors who say "the science is settled" haven't read the science. The media who claim to fact-check are just laundering press releases. And the pharmaceutical companies—the ones cashing in on all of this—have legal immunity, government protection, and zero incentive to tell you the truth.

So who's left?

You.

You, and millions of others just like you—parents, patients, physicians, scientists, and everyday citizens—who woke up one day and realized that the world of medicine isn't what it seems. That the "safe and effective" mantra doesn't hold up under scrutiny. That the injuries are real. That the data is manipulated. That the logic is broken. That the pressure is political. That the cost is human.

And still—you're standing.

Stronger, smarter, and more awake than you've ever been.

That's not crazy. That's courage.

And it's growing.

Every day, more people are stepping outside the echo chamber. They're refusing the fear. They're reclaiming their health, their autonomy, their critical thinking. They're reading the books, watching the hearings, joining the forums, attending the meetings, asking the hard questions. And most of all—they're refusing to let their children become collateral damage in a game rigged for profit.

The medical industrial complex may have the media. It may have the money. But *we* have the truth. And we're not alone anymore.

So let them scoff. Let them sneer. Let them shout "misinformation!" at every uncomfortable truth.

We'll just keep reading the fine print.

And we'll keep telling the truth.

Because when you finally see how deep this rabbit hole goes—when you finally connect the dots, see the patterns, trace the money, and understand the history—there's no going back. Not to blind trust. Not to silence. Not to compliance.

You're not crazy.

You're awake.

And you're not alone.

So now what?

Now that you know all this—*really know* it—not just the headlines, but the details, the stories, the science, the incentives, the damage, the denial... what do you do with it?

Chapter 14: Now You Know

(What are you going to do with the knowledge?)

Let's take a breath.

You made it. You made it through some of the most censored, controversial, and culturally loaded topics in modern medicine. And if you're still reading, congratulations—not because you survived the book, but because you did something most people never do: you questioned the narrative. You thought critically. You opened your eyes.

Now you know.

Now you know that the pathogenic model of health—the one that paints your body as weak and in constant need of pharmaceutical intervention—isn't the only model out there. The *salutogenic* model, the one that trusts the body, supports the terrain, and encourages resilience, is not only older but, in many ways, more logical. You've seen that the germ theory—once treated like holy writ—has cracks in its foundation, starting with Koch's very first postulate, which demands that a germ not only be found in every case of disease, but *it cannot be found in healthy subjects*. You've learned that the same germs that that are said to cause disease in many cases are also found in many people who do not become ill. And that single detail alone should have upended the entire theory—but it didn't. Why? Because the pharmaceutical industry built its empire on it.

Now you know that immunity isn't something that comes in a vial. It's something your body builds. *Natural active immunity*—the kind you develop when your body meets a germ, fights it off, and remembers it—is robust, lifelong, and empowering. Vaccines offer *artificial active immunity*, a cheap imitation at best. One that often fades, requires boosters, and comes with its own risks and side effects.

We've traded resilience for convenience—and the results speak for themselves.

Now you know the Top 10 Truths about Vaccinations. You know that:

1. **The Entire Vaccine Model Is Built on a Faulty Assumption**
   The idea that you must inject disease to prevent disease sounds scientific—until you actually look at the science. The model assumes that the body needs artificial interference to develop immunity, completely bypassing the body's own natural defenses and intelligent design. It's a model built on fear and a faulty theory, not biology. Not good science.
2. **Vaccines Don't Build Herd Immunity—They Undermine It**
   The vaccine built herd immunity argument collapses under scrutiny. The math doesn't add up, and the theory only holds any weight in the context of natural infection—not artificial, temporary immunity. Instead of protecting the herd, mass vaccination introduces dependency and chronic immune dysregulation.

3. **Vaccines Didn't Save Us from Disease—We Were Already Winning**
Historical data shows that the major declines in disease mortality happened long before vaccines were introduced—thanks to clean water, sanitation, nutrition, and public health improvements. Vaccines arrived after the victory lap and claimed the trophy.

4. **The "Safe and Effective" Mantra Is a Marketing Line—Not Science**
The safety studies are thin, the control groups are often non-existent, and the placebo standard is rarely upheld. Meanwhile, "effectiveness" is measured in money, marketing and lobbying—not real-world protection. The phrase is repeated endlessly because it works—not because it's true.

5. **Vaccines Can—and Do—Cause Serious Harm**
Injury and death are not rare side effects. They're listed right on the inserts. The government has paid out billions in damages to victims through the Vaccine Injury Compensation Program—yet somehow, you're still told "it's rare." The reality is, vaccine injury is underreported, under-acknowledged, and tragically common.

6. **There's Big Money Behind Every Shot**
The vaccine industry is worth billions annually—and it's protected by law. From pharmaceutical giants to pediatrician bonus checks, the financial incentives are massive and rarely disclosed. When profits drive policy, health takes a back seat.

7. **Your Doctor Is Supposed to Tell You More—They Usually Don't**
Informed consent isn't just a moral responsibility—it's the law. But most doctors were never taught the full story. They aren't

taught what's in vaccines, how injuries manifest, or how to recognize them. How can they inform you on something they themselves, do not know. Instead, they're trained to follow the schedule without question and pressure you to do the same.

8. **Public School Does Not Require Vaccination—Just Exemption Forms**
   Contrary to what most parents are told, there is no blanket "requirement" to vaccinate for school. Every state offers at least one form of exemption—medical, religious, or philosophical. You just have to know your rights and stand your ground.

9. **Unvaccinated Children Are Often Healthier Than Their Peers**
   Despite the media blackout, the data is there—smaller studies, parental surveys, and communities like the Amish all point to the same conclusion: unvaccinated children have lower rates of chronic illness, fewer developmental delays, and stronger natural immunity.

10. **People Who Say No to Vaccines Aren't Crazy—They're Paying Attention**
    They've read the fine print. They've questioned the narrative. They've taken the time to learn what others accept blindly. These are not fringe lunatics. They are informed, intelligent, and courageous people—just like you.

So the question becomes: what now?

What do you do with this information?

If Not Vaccines, Then What?

It's the most logical question in the world: If I don't vaccinate, then how do I protect myself or my children from disease?

The answer is beautifully simple—and profoundly ignored. It's the very thing Antoine Béchamp tried to teach the world over a century ago. Germs don't make you sick. Sickness doesn't mean your body failed. And prevention doesn't come in a syringe.

The key is the *terrain*—your internal environment. Your "built-in" immune system and it's many layers of defense. Your microbiome. Your detox pathways. Your mineral stores. Your gut. Your cells. That's where health begins and ends. And when the terrain is healthy, strong, and well-supported, disease struggles to take root.

Let's break that down into real, tangible tools—natural, time-tested, science-backed ways to boost immunity that don't come with a list of possible adverse reactions a mile long. The list of these tools can fill an entire book, but let me give you a few examples to get you started:

Vitamin D: The Natural Flu Shot

Vitamin D is not just "good for your bones." It's essential for immune regulation. Studies have repeatedly shown that people with sufficient vitamin D levels get fewer colds, flus, and respiratory infections. Some researchers have even called it "the body's own vaccine." The best part? Your body makes it—for free—when exposed to sunlight. And when the sun isn't available, high-quality vitamin D3 supplements can fill the gap. Call it sunshine in supplement form. It's simple, it's safe, and it works.[1,2,3,4]

Vitamin A: The Disease Defender

Back in the days when measles was common, doctors didn't reach for needles—they reached for cod liver oil. Why? Because it's packed with vitamin A, a powerhouse nutrient that supports the integrity of mucous membranes, reduces the severity of infections, and helps regulate the immune system. Vitamin A deficiency, not vaccination status, has been directly linked to measles complications. Want to make your child resilient? Feed them carrots, sweet potatoes, pastured butter, liver, and yes—old-fashioned cod liver oil.[5,6,7,8,9]

Vitamin C: The Unsung Hero of Immune Defense

We all know vitamin C is good for colds and flu—but did you know it's much more than just your grandmother's go-to during the sniffle season?

Vitamin C is one of the most powerful, versatile, and thoroughly studied nutrients in the immune arsenal—and yet, you'd never know that if your only source of health advice was the nightly news or your pediatrician's office. Why? Because vitamin C can't be patented, sold at $300 a dose, or mandated by a pharmaceutical company. But if you actually dig into the science, the evidence is undeniable: vitamin C is one of the most effective immune-supporting, disease-fighting tools available.

It's an antioxidant. An anti-inflammatory. An immune booster. And in high enough doses, it acts almost like a *natural antiviral.*

Dr. Fred Klenner, a physician back in the mid-20th century, used high-dose vitamin C to treat everything from polio to measles, mumps, pneumonia, and viral encephalitis. That's right—*polio*. The disease that supposedly only a vaccine could cure. His case reports are nothing short of jaw-dropping.[10,11] But because his success didn't involve a pharmaceutical product, he was largely ignored by the medical establishment.

Vitamin C works by enhancing the function of white blood cells, increasing interferon production (your body's natural virus-fighting signal), and neutralizing free radicals that can damage tissues during infection. It helps shorten the duration of illness, lessen the severity of symptoms, and prevent complications. And here's the kicker—it's safe. Extremely safe. Even at high doses.[12,13,14,15]

Ever wonder why animals don't catch colds the way we do? It's because most mammals make their own vitamin C. Humans, guinea pigs, and a few primates are the exception. We have to get ours from food or supplements—and most of us aren't getting nearly enough, especially when the immune system is under stress.

When a virus hits, your vitamin C levels plummet. Your body burns through it like gasoline on a fire. That's why taking a little "just in case" isn't the same as dosing therapeutically during illness. And again—good luck hearing this from the advertisements on TV. They'll tell you about a prescription before they ever suggest a handful of citrus.

But you're smarter than that now.

Vitamin C isn't just a helpful little helper for colds. It's a legitimate, frontline defense. A natural therapy with an impeccable safety profile and a mountain of research behind it. It may not come in a syringe with a government seal on it, but that doesn't mean it's any less powerful.

If you're looking for real immunity—lasting, functional, resilient immunity—you don't have to turn to artificial shots loaded with aluminum, formaldehyde, and viral fragments. Sometimes, the most powerful medicine comes in the form of something so simple, so overlooked, that it's almost laughable.

Until it works.

Food: Your Original Medicine

This shouldn't be radical, but for some reason it is: your immune system is built on what you eat. Sugar suppresses it. Processed food inflames it. Real, whole food supports it. Nutrient-dense diets filled with seasonal produce, healthy fats, pasture-raised meats, bone broth, raw dairy, fermented foods, and plenty of clean water do more to strengthen your immune system than any pharmaceutical ever could.

Food is the way our bodies were designed to get nutrients—*not* capsules, powders, or synthetic blends cooked up in a lab. That means your best immune-boosting medicine doesn't come in a bottle. It comes from your plate.

Your body is brilliantly engineered to break down real food, extract the vitamins, minerals, antioxidants, and phytonutrients it needs, and absorb them efficiently into your system. That's how it's supposed to work. Supplementation, by definition, should be just that—a *supplement* to an already nutrient-rich diet, not a replacement for it.

Start with food. Whole, organic, unprocessed food. Colorful fruits and vegetables. Healthy fats. Clean proteins. Foods that were alive and growing before they reached your fork. Then, *if* there's still a need—if your lifestyle, environment, or specific condition calls for more—look to natural, whole-food-based supplements as a backup. But remember: no supplement, no matter how fancy the label, can outrun a poor diet.

Colloidal Silver: The Forgotten Antimicrobial

Before there were pharmaceutical antibiotics, there was silver.

For centuries—literally thousands of years—silver has been prized for its remarkable ability to fight infection. Long before the invention of penicillin or modern antiseptics, people understood that silver had natural germ-fighting properties. Ancient Greeks and Romans stored water, wine, and vinegar in silver vessels to keep them fresh. American pioneers would drop a silver dollar into their milk jugs to delay spoilage before refrigeration. During World War I, field medics used silver-soaked gauze to dress battlefield wounds and prevent infection. They weren't guessing—they knew it worked.

But what is colloidal silver, exactly?

Colloidal silver is simply ultra-fine microscopic particles of pure elemental silver suspended in water. That's it. No additives. No synthetic chemicals. No pharmaceutical fillers. Think of it as mineral water—but with one single mineral: silver. The particles are so small (measured in nanometers) that they remain suspended in the water, creating a solution that looks like clear water, because it is clear water.

This isn't silverware. This isn't jewelry. This is silver in its smallest, bioactive form—what your body can actually use.

So, how does it work?

The science behind silver's antimicrobial action is both elegant and powerful. Silver particles have a positive electrical charge, which allows them to bind to negatively charged parts of bacterial and viral cell membranes. Once attached, the silver ions disrupt the cell wall, interfere with respiration, and penetrate the inner structures of the pathogen, causing structural and genetic damage. In bacteria, silver binds to proteins and DNA, which inhibits reproduction and halts metabolism—effectively shutting down the pathogen. In viruses, silver can prevent them from attaching to and penetrating host cells, stopping infection at the gate.[16,17,18,19,20]

In short, silver attacks germs on multiple levels. It's like a biochemical Swiss army knife—destroying bacteria, neutralizing viruses, and even eliminating some fungi. And it does all this *without creating resistant strains*. Unlike modern antibiotics, which have given rise to terrifying superbugs, silver doesn't leave behind survivors to mutate and regroup.

And here's where things get even more interesting:

Unlike today's antibiotics—which act like a wrecking ball and destroy everything in their path, including your beneficial gut flora—colloidal silver is absorbed in the upper digestive tract, before it ever reaches your good bacteria. That means it can neutralize pathogens in your system without wiping out the healthy bacteria in your gut—the very flora you need to digest food, regulate immunity, and maintain a balanced microbiome. Antibiotics often cause collateral damage. Silver doesn't. It's more like a surgical strike than a carpet bomb.[21,22,23,24]

But here's what really sets colloidal silver apart:

It's toxic to single-celled organisms—the bad guys like bacteria and viruses—but completely harmless to multicellular organisms, like you and me. Our cells are far more complex, protected by thicker membranes and immune systems that are not easily disrupted by silver particles in safe doses. In fact, small amounts of silver occur naturally in food and water, and your body can safely use it, process it, and eliminate it naturally.

Of course, as with any natural remedy, it's important to be informed and responsible. Always consult with a trusted natural health practitioner before using colloidal silver—especially when considering long-term use or treating children. Just like with vitamins or herbs, correct dosing and quality sourcing matter.

The bottom line? Colloidal silver is a time-tested, science-backed antimicrobial that has been quietly sidelined—not because it stopped working, but because it couldn't be patented. Big Pharma can't bottle it and slap a billion-dollar price tag on it, so they ignore it. But you don't have to.

And of course, as you can imagine, the FDA has not approved this message and requires the following statement: *"These statements have not been evaluated by the Food and Drug Administration. This product is not intended to diagnose, treat, cure, or prevent any disease."*

But always remember: It's your body. Your health. Your decision.

Exercise: The Forgotten Immune Booster

Want to know what stimulates lymph flow, improves circulation, detoxifies the body, reduces inflammation, and boosts white blood cell activity? Movement. Regular, moderate exercise is one of the most reliable ways to keep your immune system humming. You don't need a gym membership. Go for a walk. Stretch. Do some yard work. Ride a bike. Dance with your kids. Move your body—because stagnant bodies create stagnant immunity.

Chiropractic: Don't Miss This Part

Of all the health strategies misunderstood—and, frankly, misrepresented—by the mainstream medical world, chiropractic care sits at the top of the list. Dismissed as "just for back pain" or pigeonholed as "neck cracking," it's often treated like a fringe therapy at best, a joke at worst. But make no mistake—chiropractic isn't about your back. It's about your brain. And when you understand that, everything changes.

The entire foundation of chiropractic is built on one simple, profound truth: *the brain and central nervous system control everything in the body.* Every cell. Every tissue. Every organ. Every system—including your immune system. Your heart doesn't beat on its own. Your lungs don't decide when to breathe. Your liver, your pancreas, your digestion, your healing responses—none of it happens randomly. It's all coordinated, 24/7, by the nervous system.

The nervous system is the master control system. When the brain can communicate with the body freely and without interference, health is achievable. But when that communication is blocked, distorted, or interfered with—even slightly—malfunction sets in. And where there is malfunction, disease is not far behind.

This is where chiropractic steps in.

Doctors of Chiropractic are trained to locate and correct a very specific type of interference in the nervous system called *vertebral subluxation.* A subluxation occurs when a spinal bone becomes misaligned in such a way that it disrupts normal nerve flow. Sometimes that interference shows up as back pain or stiffness. But more often, it's silent—causing problems in digestion, sleep, hormone balance, immune function, and more.

By correcting subluxations through precise spinal adjustments, chiropractors *restore the vital communication between the brain and the body.* This allows the body to function as it was designed to: intelligently, adaptively, and healthfully. And yes—this includes your immune system.

This perspective partners beautifully with Béchamp's terrain theory. Instead of fighting germs with injections and prescriptions, chiropractic aims to strengthen the host. You don't need to sterilize the world if your internal terrain is inhospitable to disease. That's the chiropractic model. We don't build our strategy around fear of pathogens. We build it around confidence in the body.

And the results speak for themselves.

In over three decades of practice as a Doctor of Chiropractic, I've seen it again and again: families under regular chiropractic care get sick less often, bounce back more quickly, and navigate cold and flu seasons with less drama. Kids under chiropractic care often avoid the revolving door of antibiotics, inhalers, allergy meds, and urgent care visits. Adults sleep better, digest better, and function better. And the elderly retain more vitality than their drug-dependent peers.

And yes—this includes the unvaccinated. Many families who forgo vaccination include chiropractic care as a central part of their health strategy. Not just because they're looking for an alternative to shots—but because they understand something deeper: that health comes from within, not from a needle.

Chiropractic's philosophy is what separates it from traditional medicine. Medicine sees the body as a machine—replace the part, suppress that symptom, override this system. Chiropractic sees the body as an intelligent, self-healing organism, powered by something greater than just tissue and chemistry.

That "something greater" is what chiropractors refer to as Innate Intelligence.

Innate Intelligence is the inborn wisdom that animates every living being. It's what coordinates the beating of your heart, the rhythm of your lungs, the production of enzymes and hormones, the regeneration of cells, and the fighting of infection. You don't think about these things. You don't control them consciously. They just happen—perfectly, miraculously—unless something gets in the way.

And that's what subluxation does. It gets in the way. Chiropractic removes the interference and lets Innate do its job. As B.J. Palmer—the developer of chiropractic and one of the most influential health thinkers of the 20th century—once said, *"Innate Intelligence knows more in one second than man will ever know."* That's not poetry. That's reality. No doctor, no scientist, no pill can replicate the intelligence your body was born with. And no outside intervention—vaccine, drug, or otherwise—can replace it.

Another one of B.J. Palmer's insights strikes at the heart of this entire conversation. He said, *"While other professions are concerned with changing the environment to suit the weakened body, chiropractic is concerned with strengthening the body to suit the environment."*

That's it. That's the whole game.

Vaccines, antibiotics, hand sanitizers, and medical interventions all aim to manipulate the environment—to make it safer, cleaner, less threatening. But that approach never makes the body stronger. It never teaches the immune system to do its job. Chiropractic, on the other hand, is about building up the body, so it can handle whatever comes its way.

Let's not pretend chiropractic is fringe. Let's stop acting like it's alternative. It's foundational.

It's no accident that patients under regular chiropractic care report better immune function, fewer infections, faster recovery times, and greater resilience. And yes—many of those patients have chosen not to vaccinate. They're not crazy. They're not reckless. They're simply tuned into a deeper truth: when the nervous system is free of interference, and the body is supported with proper nutrition, rest, movement, and care, it is fully capable of protecting itself.

Chiropractic isn't just about spinal health. It's about life expression. It's about the full, uninterrupted function of the body's innate intelligence. And in a world constantly trying to override the body with chemicals and shots, choosing chiropractic care is a radical act of trust. Trust in nature. Trust in the body. Trust in yourself.

So if you're looking for a real alternative to vaccination—something grounded not in fear, but in empowerment—start with the nervous system. Start with chiropractic.

Because health isn't something you inject. It's something you release.

So… Now You Know. (What Are You Going to Do with This Information?)

"Each time a man stands up for an ideal, or acts to improve the lot of others, or strikes out against injustice, he sends forth a tiny ripple of hope."

— *Robert F Kennedy*

Let's pause for a moment.

You made it. Through all 14 chapters. Through all 10 truths. Through all the data, the history, the inconvenient facts, the uncomfortable realizations. You've seen the fine print. You've questioned the "settled science." You've followed the trail of logic, testimony, and real-world outcomes that led you here.

You now know more about vaccinations than most medical professionals. More than most pediatricians. More than nearly every news anchor, policymaker, or pharmaceutical rep pushing the party line. That's not arrogance—it's reality.

And now comes the most important question of all: *What are you going to do with this information?*

You cannot un-know what you now know. You can't unsee the patterns. You can't un-hear the silence that follows the cries of injured children, the warnings from whistleblowers, the data that never makes the headlines.

You've heard it all your life: "Vaccines are safe and effective." But now you know what that really means. You know how that mantra was built—on half-truths, on liability-free products, on manipulated science, on regulatory capture, on fear, and on an ever-expanding schedule that treats your children like test subjects in a billion-dollar experiment.

You've seen the truth behind the curtain.

You've learned about the difference between *the pathogenic model*—which sees your body as weak and vulnerable—and the *salutogenic model*, which recognizes that your body is intelligently designed, capable of healing, and resilient by nature.

You've seen how the germ theory crumbles under its own weight—especially under Koch's First Postulate. You've seen how modern medicine clings to a 150-year-old theory that's never truly held up to scientific scrutiny.

You've learned the difference between *Natural Active Immunity* and *Artificial Active Immunity*—and how only the former provides robust, lifelong protection, while the latter offers weak, temporary resistance at best, often at a high cost to your health.

You've heard the stories. You've seen the data.

You've walked through:

- The reality of vaccine injuries and deaths
- The legal immunity granted to vaccine manufacturers
- The unspoken influence of financial incentives

- The way public school "requirements" are really just exemption policies in disguise
- The shocking health of unvaccinated populations
- And the truth about the intelligent, thoughtful people who refuse to blindly comply

You now stand among them.

You are no longer just a passive healthcare consumer. You are informed. You are awake. You are equipped. And that makes you dangerous to the status quo.

So now the work begins.

Start by having the conversations—especially with those closest to you. This decision should be made *before* children are even conceived. However, if you already have children, it's not too late. Spouses, partners, family members—get on the same page. If you're not aligned, then dig deep and do the research together. Demand to hear both sides. Don't let anyone, not even a doctor, make life-altering decisions for your family without full informed consent.

Then get involved.

Become an advocate in your state. Learn your exemption laws. Fight to preserve them. If your state only offers medical exemptions, push to include religious and philosophical options. If your rights are threatened, speak out. Join groups. Support organizations. Educate your local legislators.

Be bold.

Speak truth in love—but speak it. Share what you know. Be the neighbor who gently plants a seed of curiosity. Be the parent who asks the uncomfortable question in the school meeting. Be the voice that breaks the illusion.

Don't wait for someone else to fight this battle. It's yours. It's your body. Your child. Your family. Your right.

Most of all—stay encouraged.

You're not alone. You're now part of a movement that stretches across every state, every country, every generation. This is not about being anti-anything. It's about being *pro-truth*, *pro-health*, and *pro-freedom*.

The generations before us didn't know what you now know. But the generations ahead are counting on you to protect their future.

So rise. Speak. Act.

Because now you know.

Chapter Sources

1. Martineau, A. R., Jolliffe, D. A., Greenberg, L., Aloia, J. F., Bergman, P., Dubnov-Raz, G., ... & Camargo, C. A. (2017). Vitamin D supplementation to prevent acute respiratory infections: Systematic review and meta-analysis of individual participant data. *BMJ, 356*, i6583.
2. Aranow, C. (2011). Vitamin D and the immune system. *Journal of Investigative Medicine, 59*(6), 881–886.
3. Cannell, J. J., Vieth, R., Umhau, J. C., Holick, M. F., Grant, W. B., Madronich, S., Garland, C. F., & Giovannucci, E. (2006). Epidemic influenza and vitamin D. *Epidemiology and Infection, 134*(6), 1129–1140.
4. Holick, M. F. (2007). Vitamin D deficiency. *New England Journal of Medicine, 357*(3), 266–281.
5. World Health Organization. (2011). *Vitamin A supplementation: A decade of progress*. WHO Press.
6. Sommer, A. (1983). Nutritional blindness, xerophthalmia, and keratomalacia. *Oxford University Press.*
7. Sommer, A., & West, K. P. (1996). Vitamin A deficiency: Health, survival, and vision. Oxford University Press.
8. Sudfeld, C. R., Navar, A. M., & Halsey, N. A. (2010). Effectiveness of measles vaccination and vitamin A treatment. *International Journal of Epidemiology, 39*(Suppl 1), i48–i55.
9. Stephensen, C. B. (2001). Vitamin A, infection, and immune function. *Annual Review of Nutrition, 21*, 167–192.
10. Klenner, F. R. (1949). The treatment of poliomyelitis and other virus diseases with vitamin C. *Southern Medicine & Surgery, 111*(7), 209–214.

11. Klenner, F. R. (1953). The vitamin and antibiotic treatment of poliomyelitis. *Journal of Applied Nutrition, 6*(3), 274–278.
12. Levy, T. E. (2011). Curing the incurable: Vitamin C, infectious diseases, and toxins (3rd ed.). MedFox Publishing.
13. Carr, A. C., & Maggini, S. (2017). Vitamin C and immune function. *Nutrients, 9*(11), 1211.
14. Hemilä, H. (2017). Vitamin C and infections. *Nutrients, 9*(4), 339.
15. Chatterjee, I. B. (1973). Evolution and the biosynthesis of ascorbic acid. *Science, 182*(4118), 1271–1272.
16. Lemire, J. A., Harrison, J. J., & Turner, R. J. (2013). Antimicrobial activity of metals: Mechanisms, molecular targets and applications. *Nature Reviews Microbiology, 11*(6), 371–384.
17. Rai, M., Yadav, A., & Gade, A. (2009). Silver nanoparticles as a new generation of antimicrobials. *Biotechnology Advances, 27*(1), 76–83.
18. Morris, J. L., Sutton, J. M., & Lian, L. Y. (2019). Silver bullets: Mechanistic aspects of metal ion antimicrobial activity and opportunities for application. *Current Opinion in Chemical Biology, 52*, 110–117.
19. Galdiero, S., Falanga, A., Vitiello, M., Cantisani, M., Marra, V., & Galdiero, M. (2011). Silver nanoparticles as potential antiviral agents. *Molecules, 16*(10), 8894–8918.
20. Lara, H. H., Ayala-Nuñez, N. V., Ixtepan-Turrent, L., & Rodriguez-Padilla, C. (2010). Mode of antiviral action of silver nanoparticles against HIV-1. *Journal of Nanobiotechnology, 8*(1), 1.
21. Drake, P. L., & Hazelwood, K. J. (2005). Exposure-related health effects of silver and silver compounds: A review. *Annals of Occupational Hygiene, 49*(7), 575–585.

22. Lansdown, A. B. G. (2006). Silver in health care: Antimicrobial effects and safety in use. *Current Problems in Dermatology, 33*, 17–34.
23. Kim, J. S., Kuk, E., Yu, K. N., Kim, J. H., Park, S. J., Lee, H. J., ... & Cho, M. H. (2007). Antimicrobial effects of silver nanoparticles. *Nanomedicine: Nanotechnology, Biology and Medicine, 3*(1), 95–101.
24. Gaul, J. (2008). *The ultimate colloidal silver manual* (2nd ed.). Life & Health Research Group.

www.ingramcontent.com/pod-product-compliance
Lightning Source LLC
Chambersburg PA
CBHW060448030426
42337CB00015B/1522